# ROLLIN' ON

# ROLLIN' ON

## A Wheelchair Guide

### to U.S. Cities

MAXINE H. ATWATER

DODD, MEAD & COMPANY

NEW YORK

1  2  3  4  5  6  7  8  9  10

Library of Congress Cataloging in Publication Data

Atwater, Maxine.
   Rollin' on.

   1. United States—Description and travel—
1960–        —Guide-books.  2. Physically handicapped—United States—Recreation.  3. Physically
handicapped—United States—Transportation.  I. Title.
E158.A85        917.3′04′926        78-15289
ISBN  0-396-07548-7

# Contents

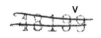

v

As a leading advocate in the removal of architectural and transportation barriers, the National Easter Seal Society for Crippled Children and Adults is delighted to see the publication of a book like *Rollin' On.*

Such a book draws new attention to how far we've come and what still needs to be done so that the wheelchair user has equal access to all of America. *Rollin' On* underlines all our efforts to broaden the world for the disabled. The book opens new vistas by showing those in wheelchairs how they can with the minimum expenditure of time and energy see the great sights in our American cities. It also dramatizes by the very feasibility of the suggested itineraries that those in wheelchairs can travel independently. The Easter Seal Society endorses this book for its basic concept that it is time for the wheelchair user to travel independently. We also endorse it for the carefully planned itineraries, the commitment to accuracy and the manner in which the advice and involvement of wheelchair leaders were sought in the featured cities. As this book heralds the new age of travel for the disabled, we also acknowledge that "the time is now" and encourage the disabled everywhere to keep rollin' on.

> —CHARLES C. CAMPBELL
> President
> The National Easter Seal Society
> for Crippled Children and Adults

Your new book *Rollin' On* for people in wheelchairs and those with other mobility limitations is an invaluable addition to furthering independent living for disabled people.

I know that some members of the President's Committee staff have worked with you in testing your new itineraries for various cities and are enthusiastic about the contribution to their lives which *Rollin' On* offers.

*Rollin' On* does more, however, than further independence. It offers a challenge to disabled people to take advantage of the numerous opportunities offered in a number of American cities, opportunities to seek work in an accessible environment.

Congratulations to you on *Rollin' On*.

> —HAROLD RUSSELL
> Chairman
> The President's Committee on Employment
> of the Handicapped

As a representative of over eleven thousand paralyzed veterans and as a disabled individual, I have long sought the publication of such a book as *Rollin' On*. Its purpose is to inform and entice the reader to venture away from the comfortable secure surroundings he already knows and experience things new and foreign to him. Travel is an enterprise that combines education, socialization, and adventure; three elements crucial to the rehabilitation of a severely handicapped person. While attaining this knowledge, this confidence and these social skills you will be imparting the same to those who previously failed to recognize the seriously handicapped individual as a real human being with normal needs and aspirations.

Travel is not always simple or easy for the ambulatory person and for one confined to a wheelchair there are times when it is a monumental task. This book will not solve all your problems but can open new horizons, ones that will create memories to last a lifetime.

—JAMES A. MAYE
Executive Director
Paralyzed Veterans of America

Travel! The word is magic to me. And a book like *Rollin' On* will make the trip easier. With it people in wheelchairs now can travel with as much certainty as any traveler can, knowing before he or she sets out what to expect at a hotel, restaurant or sightseeing attraction.

By taking the unknowns out of travel, *Rollin' On* opens a new era of adventure and independence for the mobilely disabled. Perhaps its greatest value is its challenge, its invitation to get out there and make things happen by showing the world the disabled won't be content with only an occasional outing around their own hometowns. I applaud both this challenge and the valuable information that makes wheelchair travel a reality right now!

—JILL KINMONT
*The Other Side of the Mountain*

# Acknowledgments

. . . to Bob Ruffner and Diane Lattin of the President's Committee for Employment of the Handicapped, whose early support convinced me that the time had truly come for *Rollin' On.*

. . . to Jim Maye, former director of the Paralyzed Veterans of America, and Lynn Park of the President's Committee for Employment of the Handicapped, whose spirit and humor allowed me to know that disabled people are among the most independent and fun-loving people anywhere.

. . . to my wheelchair advisers (introduced later in this book) who shared their enthusiasm and knowledge of their cities with me. And to their organizations: the Easter Seal Society of Honolulu, New York and San Antonio; Chicago's Rehabilitation Institute; Philadelphia's Mayor's Office for the Handicapped.

. . . to The National Easter Seal Society.

. . . to the Convention and Visitors Bureaus of the following cities with special thanks to the persons noted: Chicago, Bill Willis; Honolulu, Lindy Boyes; New York, Lois Elias; Philadelphia, Janet Fuhrman; San Antonio, Charles Stephens; San Diego, Al Reese; San Francisco, Cindy Westbrook.

. . . to Doug Annand, author of *The Wheelchair Traveler*, for his pioneer efforts in researching travel information for the disabled. And to Moss Rehabilitation Hospital's Travel Information Center for their service to handicapped travelers.

. . . to Dodd, Mead & Company and executive editor Allen Klots for their social consciousness and the foresight in publishing a book aimed at the mobiley disabled.

   . . . Thank you and bouquets to you for all your inspiration and assistance in getting our book out into the world!

**Introducing . . .**

*Rollin' On* advisers

- Patsy Alford, Executive Secretary, Bexar County Easter Seal Society. (See page 159)

- Aulton and Marene Aulger, San Diego. He's a leading force in the local Indoor Sports Club chapter and she teaches independent living for the handicapped. (See page 189)

- Jack Catlin, director of the Rehabilitation Institute's department of environmental advocacy, Access Chicago. (See page 53)

- John Edmonds, Chairman of the Board of Control, San Francisco Muni (Transportation), Handicapped and Elderly Study. (See page 226)

- Bonnie Gellman, Director, Mayor's Office for the Handicapped, Philadelphia. (See page 136)

- Lowell Grant, member of Mayor's Committee on Handicapped, Chairman of Barrier Free Design and Transportation, Honolulu. (See page 84)

- Eileen Healy, Office Manager, Easter Seal Society of New York. (See page 109)

- Diane Lattin, Editor, *Performance Magazine*, President's Committee on Employment of the Handicapped, Washington, D.C. (See page 265)

# Introduction

If you were a dear friend who asked me, "What shall I do when I'm in San Francisco, Chicago, or any big city?", I'd have a lot to say. Impressions would hurry to mind, some reflected from the days when I first became a tourist snug in the rumble seat of my parents' 1930-vintage Ford. Like carefully-stored treasures, the wonderful things I had discovered while traveling would clamor for expression.

"Why you must see this and that and while you're in the area, stop to see that, too. And, oh yes, if you go one block more you'll see this and behind it a fabulous view, and to its side a tiny cafe for tea and cookies. But wait there's more. See this and that too and don't forget . . ."

How could I say it all? I couldn't. That's why I've written it all down for you instead.

As I wrote I pictured you. Somehow I knew you'd enjoy the things I found interesting. Like me, I figured you'd want to see beautiful scenes, famous sites, great museums and galleries. You'd want to see and be with people, too, joining them on tours and cruises, in parks and shopping centers, in restaurants and theaters. If my hunch was right you'd also welcome the chance to get off the tourist track and get to know the city that only the residents know.

Frankly, I didn't visualize your wheelchair as much as I did you. I saw you smiling, ready for the good things, and philosophical about the unavoidable mishaps that are part of any travel adventure.

So with you in mind, I first listed my favorite things to see and do in the major cities. Then, because I wanted this book to be useful to wheelers, I checked to find out which were accessible. Surprisingly, most of the important and beautiful places turned out to be totally or partially accessible. The ones that weren't accessible I took off the list, but not that many had to go. I reminded myself that no one sees everything no matter how well they plan a trip; the things you'll miss are planned that way!

Now that I'm home again, having checked every entrance, layout and restroom personally or through a wheelchair adviser, I wish I could set out with you. How I'd like to tag along to know your experiences as you sightsee around the country. I'd like to know what you enjoy most on your visit to a city, how helpful and friendly the people are, which restaurants appeal most to you. Above all, I'd like to be with you when you adventure through a doorway and become a pioneer.

As my friend Mikki Smith in Honolulu points out, "You're going places in a wheelchair where people in chairs have never gone before. That makes you no less a pioneer than your great grandmother who crossed the prairie in a covered wagon."

But since I can't be with you, dear friend and pioneer, perhaps you can write to me, giving me the answers to those things I wonder about. You can tell me, too, how you'd like to see the itineraries changed or improved, what should be added or deleted. Your reactions and suggestions will be welcomed and put to good use when this book is revised.

So as you set out on your great travel adventure, know that you go with my best wishes for a safe and happy journey. I wish you the joy of discovery and a richness of memories. More than that, I wish you experiences that open new doors into your mind and heart. Goodbye for now, and don't forget to write!

# PART ONE

## *To Get Rollin'*

# 1

# The Time Is Now

Welcome to the revolution . . .
- the revolution of chair wheels as armchair dreamers become wheelchair travelers;
- the beginnings of a revolution in awareness as the travel industry becomes conscious of the untapped wheelchair travel market.

You are the leader who right now can help more of the barriers tumble, more ramps go up, more hotel rooms, restrooms, and restaurants be turned into accessible facilities. You can make things happen by getting out there and traveling, by showing the world that you won't be confined to your hometown or content with an occasional bus tour to a convention in a neighboring city.

Ready or not, here you come!

And surprisingly, much of the USA is ready for you. There's still a lot to do, but many hotels, restaurants, and tourist attractions in great numbers of cities offer facilities for the wheelchair traveler. There's enough out there to insure your comfort, safety, and enjoyment.

But to travel now before everything is completely ready for the wheelchair traveler requires a realistic view with respect to choosing the American cities to be visited and carefully planning the things to do and see in each.

The answers to the questions that have caused other wheelchair adventurers to stay home must be given.

You've decided to roll on out there. Already your head and heart are collaborating to choose the perfect destination. Maybe you'll

3

visit one of the eight cities featured in this book, or perhaps you'll pioneer, discovering your own special destination.

Wherever you go, you want the basic travel information that applies to almost any city, the general facts about hotels, transportation, and sightseeing. These are the raw materials from which you can fashion a trip almost anywhere in the United States. With them you'll be able to make intelligent choices, saving yourself time and trouble and avoiding disappointment.

In this section you'll get the information you need to plan your trip and to best enjoy yourself once at your destination. The chapter on "Getting Ready" tells how a travel agent can help make your vacation a success and gives a list of travel agents and tour operators specializing in travel for the mobilely handicapped. This section also gives a rundown on your transportation options, reviewing travel by air, train, bus, and car. Finally, "Getting Ready" covers the hotel picture, giving information on what you can expect at the major chains.

"On the Scene" tells you what you can expect at your sightseeing destination as far as getting inside buildings, getting around by bus and taxicab, or rolling on your own are concerned. This chapter also includes some general ideas on tipping.

Is the airport or train station accessible and will I find a usable restroom? What accessible hotels are near shops, restaurants, and attractions that I can explore on my own? Are there any special wheel-aboard buses or taxis available? Where can I go at night? Will I find accessible restrooms along the way?

After these basic questions are answered, the wheeler also has to know what are the important sights to see and what's near what. How can I see the city efficiently, for I don't have unlimited time or energy. What's near the White House, near the docks for the Statue of Liberty boat, or on the way to San Francisco's Golden Gate Park that I can also see? The wheelchair traveler also wants to know if there's a good restaurant that's accessible on San Antonio's waterfront, if he or she can lunch in the Delegates' Dining Room at the United Nations, where there's an accessible restaurant among the Chicago skyscrapers.

In addition to finding out what to see, what other sights are nearby, and what accessible restaurants are within wheelable distances, the wheelchair traveler wants to know when to see each attraction. If one visits the Chicago Art Institute on a Thursday evening, for instance, can he or she follow the visit by rolling across the street to Orchestra Hall to hear the Chicago Symphony Orchestra? The wheelchair traveler knows that if one wishes not to retrace his or her path, timing is essential.

These questions are just the beginning, however. The adventurous traveler also asks how to find the special places, those insider's restaurants that any traveler likes to talk about. Where can one see an herbalist's shop in San Francisco's Chinatown? Where can I sample Chicago's deep-dish pizza? How can I see the inside of a Fifth Avenue mansion in New York? How can I get to see the elegant diplomatic reception rooms at the Department of State in Washington?

By assessing all the accessibility information, talking with friends, studying maps and charting sightseeing courses, the devoted wheelchair traveler can come up with a probable travel adventure. But the patience, time, and energy required are almost unlimited. This book does the work instead.

*Rollin' On* answers all these questions and by doing so takes the trouble, the frustration, the fear out of wheelchair travel—and adds some magic, too.

The way the book answers the questions is unique. Instead of relating disconnected accessibility facts, *Rollin' On* fashions the information into carefully designed itineraries for each of eight cities. Sightseeing attractions are grouped by area. Convenient restaurants in or near sightseeing destinations are suggested. The best means of transportation for reaching them is offered.

The result is that with *Rollin' On* you can travel with certainty, free to concentrate your attention on beautiful scenes, great art, music, and good food instead of worrying and wondering if you'll get where you're headed—and back. Everything you'll need to know to plan your trip and to enjoy it once you arrive at your destination is here.

The suggested day-by-day itineraries for the eight cities featured in this book have been designed for both standard and electric wheelchair travelers. But because most itineraries involve the use of taxicabs, the wheelchair traveler using these itineraries must be able to lift him- or herself in and out of a taxicab or, if not, should travel with an able companion who can assist in the lifting.

The itineraries have been planned so that the standard wheelchair user can travel alone or in the company of another wheelchair companion—except for the opening of a door and calling and boarding taxicabs, no assistance is necessary.

Each daily itinerary has been planned with accessibility as the first consideration. Major sightseeing attractions that are minimally or completely inaccessible will be mentioned as options but not featured as daily itinerary destinations. Those sightseeing attractions that are featured are accessible with a notation as to which entrance to use and whether it is necessary to telephone ahead.

Accessible restrooms are a prime consideration. A list precedes each daily itinerary, indicating where the facilities especially designed for wheelchair use are located.

The restaurants suggested in the daily itineraries and listed in the "What to See and Do" portion of each city chapter can be reached without going up or down more than one or two steps. If there are stairs—even one step—they're noted.

Suggested routes almost always follow flat or almost flat terrain, with slight inclines noted. Distances for self-pushed tours are rarely over two blocks without an interesting place to stop for a rest or refreshment en route.

All sightseeing itineraries have been planned to offer a variety of experiences. On a single day the traveler may visit a museum, sip tea in an outdoor cafe, explore a famous park, sightsee from a skyscraper, and tour a shopping center. On another day he or she may take a conducted tour of an art gallery, visit a zoo, lunch at a wharfside market, cruise aboard a harbor boat, and attend a concert. Indoor sightseeing is balanced with good fresh air as the wheelchair traveler enjoys a roll down a historic trail, along a river, or through a fragrant garden.

Both dining and cultural experiences are featured in each daily itinerary. Suggestions are made for visits to restaurants that are both accessible and outstanding in ambience or culinary excellence. An effort is made to suggest a variety of dining experiences: fish chowder at a wharfside cafe, fruit salad at a garden cafe, fine French cuisine in an internationally famous restaurant, a picnic beside a boat harbor, steak and potato atop a revolving skyscraper.

Entertaining ideas for an evening include the expected and the surprising: a concert in a world-famous art gallery, libations at a off-beat jazz club, a ramble to hear lively street musicians, a play at a historic theater, an evening cruise.

Following this introductory chapter, you'll get your travel basics: information useful in all the cities included in this book. You'll find out such general information as what you can expect when traveling by air or train, what wheelchair facilities hotel chains offer, how best to get around in a city—and much more.

Each of the city chapters is organized with an introduction giving the highlights of the city, details on the best ways to get around, a recommended hotel or two, and information on preplanning the trip.

Preceding each daily sightseeing itinerary is a capsule listing of what you'll be seeing and doing, followed by a listing of how to get from one place to another. Also in this capsule is a listing of the things you'll need to know or do before setting out and details on the restrooms along the way.

At the end of the book you'll find information on other major cities and a listing of sources for further travel information.

It's all here and the time is now to get rolling into the wonderful world of travel that awaits you in U.S. cities.

The next move is yours! Let the good times roll . . .

# 2

# To Get Rollin'

Not only do you have yourself to think of, but you also have your chair. You'll want to be sure your chair is in top condition. Have it checked just before you go, with special attention to tightening all the bolts and greasing it carefully. It's also a good idea to carry insurance on the wheelchair if it isn't covered in a general policy.

Wheelchair travel experts advise taking the floor boards off the chair if it's being checked as baggage, taking along a spare axle, and carrying a tool kit for minor repairs. Always stick an identification mark on your chair.

As for yourself, be sure you have all medicines with you and not in a suitcase you'll be checking. Take along your prescriptions and an extra pair of glasses. Make a rainproof carry-all that can be hung over your wheelchair handles for shopping and sweaters. Don't take hand luggage or val packs—just one suitcase. Everyone agrees the happy traveler is the one who's traveling light.

Take just a few of your favorite clothes, making as many as possible those you can wash and drip dry. Bring something warm, something to keep you dry if it rains, and a sunhat, sunglasses, and lotion. As space permits, consider bringing a transistor radio, an alarm clock, a flashlight, soap for laundry, and portable munchies like nuts, dried fruit, and crackers. Since you won't be sightseeing every moment, remember to bring that book you've been trying to find time to read. So that you can make all your friends envious, bring your address book, buy your stamps ahead of time, and get ready to write postcards.

## Consult a Travel Agent

By consulting a travel agent, you pay nothing extra and can save time and money. Travel agents know the latest in air fare bargains, are aware of special hotel packages, and can look up information in references that are not generally available to you.

Some travel agents deal specifically with the disabled (see the list that follows), but even though not specialists in travel for the disabled, most are delighted to handle your reservations after you've made some basic decisions. By understanding what is available to you, you can work with your agent to create a perfect trip.

These are some of the tour operators and travel agents specializing in wheelchair travel:

**Evergreen Travel Service.** The original pioneer in tours for the physically handicapped, blind, or mentally retarded. The family-owned company, now in its eighteenth year of operation, offers personally conducted tours throughout the world. Mel, Betty, and Jack Hoffman have taken the disabled around the world three times, to Machu Picchu, to the South Pacific, Indonesia, North Africa, Europe, and to U.S. cities. As Betty Hoffman says, "We've ridden elephants, shot the rapids, been to the Taj Mahal, and out on a regular safari in Africa."

For information on the Evergreen tours, write to Evergreen Travel Service, 19429 44th St. West, Lynnwood, Wash. 98036; or call (206) 776–1184.

**Flying Wheels Tours.** Runs one- and two-week tours for wheelchair travelers to such destinations as Acapulco, Hawaii, the Orient, the Caribbean, and the West Coast. Owner is Judd Jacobson, a wheelchair traveler since 1957. Judd also makes individual travel arrangements. Acting as a travel agent, he reserves air space, issues tickets, makes hotel reservations, and handles all the other details of a successful trip. Write to Flying Wheels Tours, 143 West Bridge St., Owatonna, Minn. 55060; or call (507) 451–5005.

**Jack Parr Travel Service.** Specializes in overseas travel for the handicapped. Owner Jack Parr attempts to mix disabled and able on his tours. A recent offering was a cruise to Red China.

For information on upcoming trips, write to Jack Parr Travel Service, 3305A Arden Way, Sacramento, Calif. 95825; or call (916) 483-3497.

**Rambling Tours.** Specializes in tours for wheelchair travelers and those who walk slowly or with crutches or canes. Owners Murray and Ruth Fein implement two contraptions that help solve many of the problems of the handicapped traveler: a 16-inch wide wheelchair that can be steered up an aircraft aisle to the restroom, and an electrically operated lift that elevates wheelers to coach doors. Either one or both of the Feins accompanies each of their tours personally, along with a qualified staff. In the past tours have gone to the British Isles, Scandinavia, the Orient, Majorca, Spain, Portugal, North Africa, and Central America.

You can obtain a current tour book and other information by writing to the Feins at Rambling Tours Inc., P.O. Box 1304, Hallandale, Fla 33009; or call (305) 921-2161.

**Wider Worlds Travel for the Handicapped.** Operates tours only to Guatemala, modifying the standard Clark Tours of Guatemala as required. For information write to Wider Worlds Travel, 331 Madison Ave., New York, N.Y. 10017; or call (212) 867-6633.

### Transportation Options

New regulations and a raised consciousness on the part of the transportation industry are greatly expanding the options open to the wheeler on the move.

#### By Air

The sky's the limit, or almost, when it comes to air travel for wheelchair users. Except for travel by private automobile, there are probably fewer barriers to overcome when traveling by air than any other mode of transportation. Part of this happy fact is due to the May 1977 decree by the Federal Aviation Administration requiring all airlines to accept as many physically handicapped passengers as possible on flights and to establish procedures for assisting handicapped passengers in case of emergency. Since this decree the airlines now must include their procedures for handling the handicapped in their published tariffs. What this means is that wheelchair users traveling alone no longer can be denied passage on the grounds that they would be unable to leave the plane unaided in the event of an emergency.

The airlines are complying with the ruling as evidenced by the answers to a questionnaire sent to ten national airlines by the New York Department of Consumer Affairs in preparation of their *Consumer Rights for Disabled Citizens* booklet. Seven of the ten responded that they accept disabled passengers traveling alone with no requirement for medical certificate except in case of illness. They also reported that the airlines offer special seat assignments and diets to those who make their request ahead of time, and make airport wheelchairs for boarding and deplaning available.

The three airlines that failed to respond to the original New York Department of Consumer Affairs questionnaire have since joined the group.

As encouraging as this good news is, it's still wise to keep in mind that airlines have policies that govern the number of physically handicapped persons that can fly aboard a single plane— based on the number of exits and able crew available for assistance during emergencies. Policies at times fluctuate, with decisions up to pilots or station managers at times, so you travel with a small element of risk if you don't do as the airlines suggest—tell the ticket agent or your travel agent when you make your reservation that you are in a wheelchair and spell out what special needs you might have.

The fine TWA brochure "Consumer Information about Air Travel for the Handicapped" sums up the point:

> The most important conversation you can have affecting your journey is with the reservation agent at the time you book your flight or with your travel agent. . . . that's the time to make known your needs and to explain your particular disability so we can best serve you.

By doing so, you help the airlines communicate your needs to all the employees who will be working for you, from reservation through ticketing and finally at the airport and even your arrival destination.

The same advice is echoed by the Travel Information Service of the Moss Rehabilitation Center in this checklist of things to do to insure a smooth trip:

✔ When you book an airline ticket, tell the reservation clerk what your disability is and your needs.

✔ Double check with the airport to make sure a wheelchair is available if you require it.

✔ Make certain your airline has notified its personnel at your destination that you will need assistance in deplaning.

✔ If you are travelling alone, carry a letter from your doctor stating you are healthy enough to do so.

✔ Travel light—don't be burdened by needless possessions.

✔ Put a luggage tag on your wheelchair. Check it and your baggage through to your final destination.

✔ Use an airport wheelchair to get to and from the plane; remember, though, no wheelchair is left aboard for use in flight.

✔ Arrive at the airport early; you'll probably be the first aboard and the last off.

✔ Use a toilet in the airport terminal to avoid the lavatory on board, a cubbyhole that wasn't intended for the disabled.

✔ If your spouse must assist you in the toilet, use facilities in the terminal's first-aid stations or nursery.

✔ Tip skycaps well; this makes travel easier for those who follow you.

✔ Keep in your pocket or purse any medication you can't do without for 24 hours—just in case your luggage goes astray.

✔ Have generic names of your drugs in the event of loss or breakage—also, your physician's dosage instructions. Carry an ample supply of medication to last throughout your trip.

Air travel information worth writing for: *Air Travel for the Handicapped*, TWA Sales Dept., 2 Penn Plaza, New York, N.Y. 10010.

### Airport Accessibility

You're catching a plane or arriving at your destination airport. The important question now is "what can I expect as to the accessibility of the airport terminal?" Thanks to the *Access Travel* guide to the accessibility of airport terminals, most accessibility questions can now be answered before you arrive at your airport. The brochure is the result of an Airport Operators Council International survey of its members conducted with technical assistance from the Architectural and Transportation Barriers Compliance Board. Over 200 international airports—142 of them in the United States—are represented. Each responded to seventy-two accessibility questions that cover everything from handicapped parking facilities and car rental agencies offering hand-controlled vehicles to the slope of ramps and the size of restroom stalls. Although the accessibility of a restroom or parking facilities will probably not determine whether or not you fly to Miami or San Francisco, having the information that the brochure provides will help you make your plans and travel with greater certainty.

This *Access Travel* information is readily available to your travel agent since it's been reprinted in the Bible of the industry, the *Official Airline Guide Travel Planner & Hotel/Motel Guide*. In the Spring of 1978 this information also includes a section on airport buses and limousines with wheelchair lifts. Because of the newness of this service, it's best to doublecheck via your travel agent, especially if you are going to Chicago, Denver, New York, or San Francisco. These four cities have indicated they are currently operating wheel-aboard airport limousine services.

For your own copy of the twenty-page *Access Travel: A Guide to Accessibility of Airport Terminals*, send your request to the Consumer Information Center, Pueblo, Colorado 81009.

### By Train

The *all* in "all aboard" can include wheelers these days, thanks to new developments at the nation's major passenger railway service, Amtrak. In 1977 Amtrak began including one accessible car on each of its Amfleet trains. By the end of the year 122 accessible cars were regular features on the Amfleet runs linking eastern cities, as well as New York to Savannah, Chicago with Detroit, St. Louis and New Orleans, and on the western run between Seattle and Portland, and Los Angeles and San Diego. The one accessible car on each train features food service restrooms with both lateral and horizontal grab bars, 30-inch wide aisles, swivel seats with removable arm rests, and spaces for wheelchairs for those who cannot transfer to the train seats.

In addition to the accessible cars on the Amfleet trains, Amtrak in 1978 introduced the first of their new double-decker Superliners. These long-distance passenger trains include sleeping-car rooms designed especially for the handicapped, special seating, and restrooms. The Superliner service runs between Chicago and Seattle, with more trains planned for the San Francisco–Chicago, Chicago–Los Angeles, New Orleans–Los Angeles, and Los Angeles–Seattle runs.

Great as these new accessible trains are, the wheeler still faces one problem: the 51-inch gap between the train platform and the railroad car. Except in Washington, Philadelphia, and New York, low platforms combined with high car entrances make assistance necessary. To bridge the gap, Amtrak tries to provide assistance at the stations with low platforms. At the time you make your reservation, you'll be told if someone will be available to assist you on and off the train. This means that for the wheeler traveling between Washington, Philadelphia, and New York it's "all aboard." If you're going to other cities served by Amfleet or Superliner, it's only "all aboard" if Amtrak personnel are available to lift you on and off, or if you bring your own assistance.

For more information on Amtrak's handicapped service, write for their booklet *Access Amtrak*, c/o the Public Affairs, Amtrak, 400 N. Capital Street N.W., Washington, D.C. 20001.

### By Bus

As far as conventional airport limousines, Trailways, and Greyhound Lines buses are concerned, there's no way to "leave the driving to us" unless you can board the bus and sit in regular coach seats. But if you can, Greyhound offers an innovative "Helping Hand Service" that lets you and an able friend travel on the cost of a single ticket. In effect, you're each paying half fare. Since the aisles of the Greyhound buses are 14 inches, you probably won't be able to use the restrooms aboard, so you'll have to plan your trip carefully to permit restroom stops at those terminals that have accessible restrooms.

Write for *Helping Hand Service for the Handicapped*, Greyhound Lines, Greyhound Tower, Phoenix, Arizona 85077. For more immediate information on this special service, call your Greyhound Lines terminal and ask for the Helping Hand Service phone number.

### By Car

Some cities are car cities, others aren't. Many wheelchair travelers agree that to best enjoy Denver, Phoenix, Chicago, San Diego or Honolulu cars can come in mighty handy. If you're not driving your own, renting a car can be as practical as it is convenient. Costs vary, of course, with the type of car rented and the city where it is rented. The weekly rate is proportionally lower than the daily rate, and often weekend packages are available.

When making your plans for a "car city," you can check with a number of agencies, among them the big three: National, Avis and Hertz. Each of these offers hand-control-equipped autos at no extra cost. The type of car will vary, as will the lead time you'll need in assuring delivery of a hand-controlled vehicle. Generally, allow at least two weeks when ordering a hand-controlled car from Avis, ten days from Hertz and as little as forty-eight hours from National. To be sure you get what you want when you want it, all companies stress the importance of letting them know your plans as soon as possible. One wheeler who was rented a big car without power brakes warns you to ask for power brakes if you want them and don't just assume you'll be getting them.

At Hertz you'll have to complete an application and leave a cash deposit for the vehicle plus an additional $25 for the hand controls. National and Avis do not require an additional deposit for hand controls. All accept major credit cards.

What kinds of cars can you rent? National offers new Chevrolet Monte Carlo and Oldsmobile Cutlass two-doors. Hertz makes hand controls available on its standard sedans, such as Ford LTDs. At Avis hand controls can be attached to almost any type of rental car.

Where can you rent a hand-controlled car? If it's a Hertz car, you'll find airport rental locations at Los Angeles, San Francisco, Chicago O'Hare, Boston, Miami, Dallas/Fort Worth, Atlanta, Washington National, and Detroit Metro. Hand-controlled cars are also available in Manhattan at Hertz's East 48th Street location.

With forty-eight hours notice, National offers hand-controlled vehicles in Phoenix, Los Angeles, San Francisco, Washington, Miami, Atlanta, Chicago, Detroit, Minneapolis–St. Paul, and Houston. With more lead time National can make hand controls available in other cities.

Avis makes hand controls available in most major U.S. cities, including all those listed in this book—except San Antonio.

Many car rental companies participate with airlines and tour operators in fly/drive packages. It's always a smart idea to ask what the latest packages are.

If you're driving your own vehicle, you may find some useful information in the new American Automobile Association booklet aimed at the handicapped traveler, *The Handicapped Driver's Guide*. Request it from your local AAA office.

### The Hotel Picture

With so many hotels accessible these days, it's getting so you can choose any two or three that most appeal to you and then with a letter or phone call discover that at least one offers wheelchair-accessible facilities.

Accessibility as related to hotels means level or ramped access into the hotel and its public rooms, handicapped parking spaces, and doors at least 32 inches wide. When a guest room is designated as being especially designed for the handicapped, it generally includes hooks for pulleys over the bed, a bathroom door at least 28 inches wide, grab bars by the toilet and in the tub, a shower curtain instead of a glass door, and an extra-low sink.

Unless otherwise noted, the hotels featured in this book offer rooms especially designed for the wheelchair traveler. When a hotel is mentioned that does not offer these special rooms, a notation is made as to the width of the bathroom door.

As for hotels in other cities, here are some general facts that will aid you and your travel agent in making the best hotel choice:

Most wheelers agree that if you're staying in the heart of a city, your best bets are probably Hyatt, Hilton, Sheraton, or Western hotels. If you're driving and staying on the fringe of a city, it's probably Howard Johnson, Quality Inn, or Marriott. Holiday Inn, with properties both in the city hub and on the fringe, is also a good bet.

Some Hyatt hotels feature rooms that are especially designed for wheelchair guests. A listing of the hotels that do is being prepared by the hotel chain and should be available. For a copy write to the Public Relations Director, Hyatt Corporation, P.O. Box 945, Burlingame, California 94010.

Although Hilton Hotels doesn't list rooms especially designed for wheelchair travelers, their facilities are almost always accessible. Guest rooms feature 30-inch wide doors and lower-than-average basins. They do *not* offer conventional grab bars.

The Sheraton Corporation is at present compiling a list of wheelchair accessible facilities. To get their list, write to the Public Relations Director at The Sheraton Corporation, 470 Atlantic Ave., Boston, Massachusetts 02210.

The Western International Hotels now has a corporate policy of "exploring the possibility of making accessibility changes," and already some of the hotels are accessible, but each must be checked individually—there is no listing.

Howard Johnson's facilities offer many wheelchair-accessible guest rooms. Write for their directory c/o Public Relations, Howard Johnson's, 222 Forbes Road, Braintree, Massachusetts 02184.

Quality Inns offer wheelchair facilities in eighty cities, generally not the largest cities. For a list of facilities for wheelchair travelers, write to Quality Inns, 90750 Columbus Pike, Silver Spring, Maryland 20901.

The Marriott chain offers limited numbers of wheelchair accommodations at each of its hotels. All hotels are accessible, with ramp for entry, wide doors, handrails in bathrooms, and accessible restaurants and coffee shops.

Granddaddy of the wheelchair-accessible chains is probably Holiday Inn, which in 1966 began requiring at least one specially designed room in each new hotel for the mobilely handicapped.

About half the Holiday Inns across the country now offer accessible rooms. For a lisiting of all Holiday Inns from which you can find those with handicapped facilities, write to Public Relations, Holiday Inns Inc., 3796 LaMar Ave., Memphis, Tennessee 38118.

### Making Reservations

When making reservations, keep in mind that all these hotels have only a certain number of wheelchair rooms. To be sure of reserving one, you'll have to give the hotel plenty of notice. It's never too early to make a reservation for these special rooms, and as more and more wheelers travel, good lead time will become more important. Of course, as the hotels find their wheelchair rooms being used, more will be added.

When making your reservation, advise the hotel as to your needs. How wide is your wheelchair? Do you need grab bars? Would you like runners put down on the plush carpet? Ask and you shall receive—or at least every effort will be made to see that you get what you need.

Also ask if the hotel offers any special packages. Sometimes you can get a special rate or such bonuses as cocktails, meals, and tickets to sightseeing attractions by buying a package. Packages are usually based on double occupancy and are for two or three nights, sometimes during the week and at other times on weekends.

If, for any reason, you're not working with a travel agent, here are the toll free numbers for some of the hotel chains:

Howard Johnson (800) 654–2000
Marriott (800) 228–9290
Western International (800) 228–3000
Sheraton (800) 325–3535

For the others, call the hotel listed in your phone directory and ask for Out-of-Town Reservations.

# 3

# On the Scene

Once you've arrived at your chosen U.S. city, how will you get around? And when you finally get to that historic site, museum, or famous restaurant, will you be able to get in? What can you expect as to accessibility?

The answers to these questions vary city by city. They are given for you here very specifically for eight of the most popular cities. As for the others, the specific answers are only partially available through the "Access" books. (See the last chapter for a listing of available Access booklets and where you can obtain them.) Most answers come from people like you who communicate their travel experiences in magazine and newspaper articles, by talks to groups, and by providing information for books like this one.

Here are some of the findings of wheelers around the country:

## Seeing the Sights

As you probably know, the 1968 Architectural Barriers Act requires all public facilities built after 1968 with federal funds to be accessible to the disabled. The fuzzy wording of the regulations, however, has permitted less than total accessibility in some instances. But things are improving as the Architectural and Transportation Barriers Compliance Board finally completes its staffing and begins to move along with uniform systems for making the government agencies comply. The Board, made up of top-level representatives drawn from nine federal agencies, is now establishing a comprehensive system of compliance and setting up a self-checking system of appraisal. For this task and others it solicits the advice and recommendations of a consumer advisory panel made up of a majority of handicapped people.

Most widely used among the federal agencies and public and private concerns are the well-known American National Standards Institute (ANSI) of accessibility. Whenever you see the international symbol of accessibility you can expect that an effort has been made to comply with the ANSI or other standards of barrier-free design. But the symbol does not always mean the building actually is barrier-free and accessible; since the use of the symbol is not regulated, non-federal businesses can use it without restriction. Of course, if the symbol is misused it's probably through ignorance as to what exactly it implies.

But generally you can count on these standards of accessibility if the symbol is used: the door opens to a clear width of at least 32 inches, there are no protruding thresholds, and if the entrance is not at ground level it is reached by a gently sloping ramp. You can expect also, if the building is intended to be used for more than a half hour at a time, that you'll find accessible restrooms, telephones, water fountains, and food service.

When it comes to restrooms bearing the symbol, you can expect doors at least 32 inches wide that open out, and one stall at least 3 by 5 feet with handrails.

Wheelers everywhere chorus the refrain "speak up." If you find an attraction, restroom, restaurant, or hotel inaccessible when it bears the symbol, have the manager called, telephone him, or write a letter explaining why you could not use the facility. Register your constructive criticism. Nice letters and phone calls that don't criticize as much as they point out have done wonders.

If the inaccessible building you encounter is a federal building, take time to write a letter of complaint to the Architectural and Transportation Barriers Compliance Board, Washington, D.C. 20201. In your letter give the name of the federal agency, the address, the exact nature and location of the barrier-related problem, and the name and telephone number of the building manager. You can also offer your suggestion for solving the problem.

## Getting Around

### Bus Stop

The Transbus program signed into law on May 19, 1977, makes it mandatory for federally financed buses built after September 30, 1979, to kneel to 18 inches above the ground and to be equipped with a ramp for wheelchair boarding. Some of these new buses are already in operation in San Diego and Atlanta, and one hundred twenty lift-equipped buses have been ordered by Washington, D.C., to be in operation by the summer of 1978. The subway architects in San Francisco and Washington have also taken the wheelchair traveler into account. Both systems feature elevators that convey the wheeler to platforms and trains that include special wheelchair spaces.

In other cities, like San Diego and San Antonio, the city provides wheel-aboard vans available by reservation at nominal per ride charges. Special wheel-aboard Yellow Cab taxicabs are becoming available in some cities, and some airports now offer wheelchair limousines (a listing of these airport limousines is included in the Spring 1978 issue of the *Official Airline Guide's Travel Planner*, which is available to travel agents).

### Taxicab Tactics

In most cities, the taxicab remains the least expensive option for the wheeler who can lift himself in and out of the cab or who has assistance. Wheelers generally agree that the best way to hail a cab is by telephone. The consensus of wheelers says *not* to mention you're in a wheelchair. All agree that the cabbie should get a generous tip for the extra effort he goes to in folding and unfolding the chair and helping the wheeler in and out of the cab. If you're forced to hail a cab on the street, one wheeler advises "signal the cab like you expect it to stop for you; raise your hand high, whistle, look self-sufficient." Another wheeler has a thing for Checker Cabs, explaining that they're roomier and classier. Since the back seat is set back a little and is not even with the door you can't slide in as you can with other cabs, however; so to use a Checker Cab you'll have to know your maneuverability limitations.

### On Your Own

Rolling around the city on your own becomes more and more feasible as cities continue to cut ramps into curbs. Included in the 1973 Federal Highway Act was a mandate that after July 1976 new or renovated sidewalks be ramped. In addition, some cities have inaugurated separate programs and allocated special funds to programs aimed at cutting ramps at existing intersections regardless of whether they are being renovated or not. Progress is heartening. The city you had difficulty in yesterday could be a breeze tomorrow.

As one wheelchair traveler points out, however, "anyone in a chair who moves around has to learn to handle curbs or to ask for help. That seems to be part of the trip, at least for the present."

Of course, it helps to know what the curb cut situation is so that you won't be surprised. Since the information is hard to come by (unless you have a friend to ask), one enterprising wheeler hit on this trick: "Before you get out of the cab, take a few minutes to drive around so you can see where the curb cuts are, noting the names of the street intersections. Then at your leisure, in a park or cafe, consult your map, mark the curb cut intersections and plot your course."

### Tipping Know-how

Many people are concerned about tipping, never quite knowing if they have overdone it or tipped too little. As a general rule nowadays, tip the waiter or waitress serving you in a restaurant 15 percent. Give the taxicab driver the same—more if he goes out of his way to assist you. Since the doorman at your hotel can be your best friend, calling cabs, helping you in and out, carrying your packages into the hotel, tip him each time he gives you a hand. Fifty cents to a dollar is appropriate, depending on how much he goes out of his way for you.

One wheeler sums it up nicely: "Remember that you are asking busy people to assist you in ways that are out of the ordinary. You must give concrete expression of your gratitude, and nothing is more concrete than a couple of big chunks of silver."

# PART TWO

## *Cities to See Now*

# 4

# Deciding Where to Go

How do you decide what city to see? Is it the one you're ready for or the one that's ready for you? Do you go when it's become almost totally accessible, or do you set out like an adventurer to find what's there?

Obviously the answer depends on your nature—whether you want a breeze or a challenge, whether you're for comfort or adventure. Both are there and most often you'll get something of each, because whenever you travel you face the excitement of the unknown and, conversely, the pleasure of the familiar.

To suit both inclinations, this book has asked two questions of the most popular sightseeing cities:

- Is it relatively accessible to wheelchair travelers?
- If it isn't, is it too important to ignore?

More than a dozen cities came hurrying to mind. Some of them are included in the "Other Cities" chapter. Of all of them, eight stood out after careful research as being the cities to see now. These are Chicago, Honolulu, New York, Philadelphia, San Antonio, San Diego, San Francisco, and Washington. The reason for their inclusion?

**Chicago** because it is too important to ignore. At first glance it might seem inaccessible, particularly if you only look at the downtown Loop area. As it turns out, "the second city" boasts a surprisingly progressive attitude concerning barrier-free architecture and curb cuts. Chicago turned out to be quite accessible and filled with must-see sights. It may surprise you.

**Honolulu** had to be in the book because so many people dream of seeing it and hope it will also be a wheeler's paradise. As it turned out, Honolulu is one of the most accessible cities, with the country's only wheel-aboard taxicab and almost totally accessible sightseeing.

**Philadelphia** was chosen for both its historic importance and for its good accessibility. The major sightseeing area, the old city, got a $100 million facelifting for the Bicentennial, including ramped walkways and entrances to most of the historic buildings. The result is a compact and accessible sightseeing destination that's hard to beat.

**New York** like Chicago is too important to ignore. But unlike Chicago it turns out to be one of the least progressive of the cities when it comes to curb ramps and accessible tourist sites. However, it still offers a great deal that can be seen and enjoyed by the wheeler who has assistance—or who can get up and down curbs. Careful research and testing has made this challenge of a city a realistic destination for a wheeler.

**San Antonio** is included because every travel book has to have one exciting new discovery. San Antonio's charm, friendliness, and growing accessibility make it an upstart contender for the list of great wheelchair travel cities.

**San Diego** is an obvious addition, already with a strong reputation as a great resort city and with progressive accessibility attitudes. It's better than imagined, with diverse sightseeing, waterside walkways for rambling, and memorable bayside restaurants.

**San Francisco** demanded inclusion because of the way most people feel about this romantic city. Research provided a way to present the city of hills without an uphill climb. As it turns out, most of the major sights lie on almost flat terrain, which can be approached by the new totally accessible subway or by taxicab.

**Washington** was chosen for its superb accessibility and its historical and cultural interest. The capital's new subway system can be used for almost all sightseeing if one stays at a hotel adjacent to one of its stations. The capital could well be the United States' number-one wheelchair-accessible sightseeing city.

As you read the descriptions and detailed day-by-day itineraries of these eight great wheeler cities, picture yourself on location. Envision the things you'll see and do, choose your city and go. Even if the cities aren't completely ready for you and your wheels, *you're ready for the city* and that's all that really matters.

# 5

# Chicago

When it comes to elegance, few cities outshine Chicago. Probably nowhere else in the United States can the careful traveler revel in more luxurious surroundings, see more awe-inspiring buildings, visit richer museums, or enjoy a more bountiful greensward of parks and waterfront walkways. For a city with a reputation for "big shoulders" and as "hog butcher to the world," the news that Chicago is oozing with elegance may come as a surprise. But elegant it is—you simply have to know where to look.

Fortunately, any tourist on the beaten track sees Chicago's gold-plated portion with ease, as most of it is within the north-south rectangle that borders Lake Michigan. Within this three-mile segment of the 274-square-mile city reigns a fantasy of marble, chrome, and glass and steel buildings bordered by flower-strewn boulevards and lush waterfront parklands. The famed "Gold Coast," where once Chicago's elite maintained impressive mansions, now is a swath of posh apartment houses and condominiums. The "Magnificent Mile," stretching along North Michigan Avenue between the Chicago River and Oak Street has never been more lavish.

Basic to this elegant mien is Chicago's history of city fathers who fostered distinctive building. Here modern architecture was born, the Chicago School spawned, the first skyscraper built in 1886. Few cities boast more distinguished buildings, whether for their stylish ornamentation, sheer height, or innovative design. Styles range from Louis Sullivan's lavishly detailed Auditorium Building and the gingerbread-ornate Wrigley Building to the prototype circular Marina City and the black aluminum Sears Tower, tallest structure in the world.

In the 1950s and 1960s, Chicago became famous for one of the most ambitious urban renewal programs in the United States. Hundreds of acres of slums were cleared, and in their place a new kind of skyscraper evolved, a multi-use urban tower that combined office space with living space.

The most elegant example of this futuristic urban city-within-a-city style is the seventy-four-story Water Tower Place, a hotel, shop, restaurant, theater, and condominium complex; the one hundred-story John Hancock Center office and apartment building rivals it.

Seeing these innovative structures becomes one of the most important reasons for visiting Chicago and the easiest one to pursue, since some part of the colossal skyline is usually in view or one of its spectacular buildings at hand. Even in Lincoln Park, with its tall old hawthorne trees, the skyline dominates, growing above the green fringe like a giant rocky crystal garden.

For the wheelchair traveler the skyline of buildings can be surveyed from the waterside vantage of the Navy Pier that pokes its narrow arm 3000 feet into Lake Michigan, from the rooftop deck of Sears Tower, or from the revolving restaurant and lounges that headline the city. The broad, flat walkways that skirt Lake Michigan for miles also make ideal points from which to view the city skyline—or to cast a line with the hope that a cohoe salmon will give a nibble.

For many the idea that Chicago is a place to go fishing or rambling along a waterfront walkway might seem surprising. But Lake Michigan, the city's watering place and its reason for being, makes a beautiful playground, one that is maximized by the extensive parks that border it.

The beautiful waterfront, the swath of posh apartment houses, the incomparable sweep of skyscrapers, the gemlike shopping malls of marble and glass—it's all there. Elegance reigns and you're about to find it for yourself.

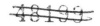

## Planning Your Trip

Even though Chicago is a more manageable city than New York, less hectic and more human, you'll still never forget you're in the nation's second largest city, with 3½ million inhabitants.

Because of its size, the pace, and the crowds, some travelers can be overwhelmed. With careful planning, however, one can with a minimum of effort see and enjoy the best that the city offers.

Begin by writing for the unusually detailed selection of information brochures offered by the Chicago Convention and Tourism Bureau, 332 South Michigan Avenue, Chicago, Illinois 60604. If you're driving or renting a car, you'll find the map available free from the Department of Transportation excellent; write to them c/o State of Illinois, Springfield, Illinois 62706.

Even if you've never developed an interest in architecture, a trip to Chicago provides a great reason to give it a try. Chicago may be America's architectural capital; at least it's a rare living textbook of architectural styles by some of the world's most renowned architects. Any book you pick up on U.S. architecture will include some of the structures you'll be seeing in Chicago. If nothing else, you can get a crash course on the most outstanding features of the major buildings by writing for the booklets published by the Commission on Chicago Historical and Architectural Landmarks, 320 North Clark St., Chicago, Illinois 60610. Ask for *The Astor District* and *Chicago Landmarks* booklets. Enclose 50¢ for each book ordered.

As second city, Chicago also boasts a lively cultural scene. Broadway plays are staged at six theaters, four of which are accessible to wheelchairs: the Arie Crown Theatre at McCormick Place, the Drury Lane Theater at Water Tower Place, the Blackstone Theater in the Loop, and the Civic Theater at Wacker and Madison streets. Operas and concerts are presented at the accessible Chicago Opera House and Orchestra Hall, circuses at Medinah Temple.

One good way to get a listing of the concerts, plays, and other cultural events to be staged during your stay is by writing to the Chicago Council on Fine Arts, 123 West Madison Avenue, Chicago, Illinois 60602. Enclose a stamped, self-addressed envelope. When you're in town you can dial F-I-N-E-A-R-T and get a recorded list of events. Make reservations by calling or writing to the theater.

Just for fun, and to whet your appetite in more ways than one, you may want to write to *Chicago Magazine*, 500 North Michigan Avenue, Chicago, Illinois 60611, requesting a current copy; enclose $1.50. This award-winning city magazine has begun noting wheelchair accessibility of tourist attractions, theaters, and restaurants. Keep in mind, however, that accessibility is defined by the person who owns or manages the attraction. To be sure, when in doubt, nothing beats a phone call with a friendly question or two.

For the latest listing of wheelchair-accessible facilities, enclose $1 and write for the current copy of *Access Chicago*, Rehabilitation Institute of Chicago, 345 East Superior Street, Chicago, Illinois 60611.

When should you go to Chicago? Summer is the only time to go, for in early June and July you'll have your best chance to enjoy the city's six to eight weeks of cool, clear days minus the fog and smog. Also, during this period you'll be on hand for the free musical events put on by the Park and Recreation Department, including concerts at the Grant Park Music Shell, Pioneer Square, and Buckingham Fountain.

As for what to take along, pack a raincoat, sunglasses, and a hat to protect you from the sun. Since you may find a dearth of food stores in the main tourist areas, it may be advisable to bring along a few nibbles from home.

## How to Get There

Chicago leads the country as number one transportation center. It is the hub of Amtrak and O'Hare International Airport is the world's busiest airport.

Chicago's Union Station is served by Amtrak. Although there are only stairs and escalators at the Canal Street entrance, ticket office and trains are level to the Clinton Street entrance. Access to restrooms is level, but stalls are not equipped for wheelchair users.

The Greyhound Bus Terminal at North Clark and West Randolph streets is accessible via the 67 West Lake Street entrance, with standard restrooms on the concourse level.

Modern Chicago O'Hare International Airport, located eighteen miles from the Loop, is one of the most accessible anywhere. The three main terminals all have ramps, automatic doors, and restrooms especially designed for wheelchair users on the upper and lower levels. For a copy of the *Airport Guide for the Handicapped & Elderly*, write to the Department of Aviation, Room 1111, City Hall, Chicago, Illinois 60602.

## Getting Around

Hooray for Chicago! Curb ramps are blossoming, and that's worth a hooray because some of those other big cities are back in the curb-ramp Dark Ages. You'll find the portion of North Michigan between the Wrigley Building and Oak Street pretty well cut, with new ones being added.

Unlike some other cities, Chicago has two programs for curb ramps: one calls for curbs to be cut whenever old streets are renovated or new ones built. The second program has earmarked $4 million in federal funds to be used to tear up existing sidewalks so curb ramps can be added. In 1977, Chicago was one of the only cities devoting its federal public works allotment entirely to a curb ramp program. In addition, under a five year plan, Chicago will spend $40 million for programs to increase the mobility of the elderly and disabled, including the addition of twenty-eight accessible subway stops. As one wheeler says, "It looks like they mean it and won't stop now until the city is one hundred percent curb ramped."

In 1976 the mayor created a separate division for the handicapped as the culmination of a progressive attitude regarding the disabled. Even before that, access for the handicapped was mandatory for any new Chicago public building, whether it was a federal building or not.

"The city of Chicago's amendments to the building code, on the books in 1973, were considered models because they made it mandatory even for renovated buildings to be accessible," says Jack

Catlin, director of the Rehabilitation Institute's department of environment advocacy, Access Chicago.

Right now what all this means is that newer buildings are accessible whether they're federal or not. It means the wheeler can roll along partially ramped North Michigan Avenue and elsewhere, and look forward to the day very soon when the Loop's high curbs will be cut, opening that interesting area.

When not rolling along North Michigan Avenue the wheelchair traveler can use the city's good taxicab service, which at 85¢ for the first one-tenth mile and 10¢ for each additional one-fifth mile isn't bad.

Another option, of course, is to rent a car with hand controls. The big three—Avis, Hertz, and National—all rent these (see Chapter 2 for details).

## Where to Stay

By locating yourself in the heart of the near north Magnificent Mile area, you'll have pushable access to a variety of shops, restaurants, and nighttime activities. Besides, you'll be in the center of Chicago's most elegant area. You'll also be ideally situated for taxi sightseeing excursions to the tourist attractions that lie outside the North Michigan Avenue cache of delights.

Choosing your hotel with accessibility and location in mind then means a decision between these top contenders:

The **Holiday Inn**–Chicago City Centre, 300 East Ohio Street, is the least expensive of the bunch and is only two blocks from either Lake Shore Drive or North Michigan Avenue. You can't compare it to most Holiday Inns you've seen. Its skylit lobby is filled with modern paintings, plants, futuristic lighting, and sensuous furniture. The hotel is really a resort, as it adjoins a complete sports center with pool and sauna and a complex of shops plus motion picture theater.

The 150-room **Tremont Hotel** off North Michigan Avenue at 100 East Chestnut was recently updated to the tune of $6 million, but it still retains its old-world charm. Highpoint is the lobby, which is more like a cozy—and very classy—living room. The walls are paneled in golden oak, the ceiling is beamed, there's a fireplace and a wealth of antiques, including a magnificent Queen Anne desk, sideboards, chests, and map table. The rooms, furnished with great style, include ones with bathroom doors that are 27 inches wide with grab bars. Adjoining the hotel is Cricket's Restaurant, managed by New York's 21 Club. Whether you stay at the Tremont or not, you may want to visit this new, rustic restaurant that features such unusual dishes as hot cabbage salad and chicken hash served with sauce mornay and wild rice.

The **Continental Plaza,** 909 North Michigan Avenue, is an elegant but expensive hotel with some wheelchair-accessible rooms, and so is the **Drake Hotel** at East Lake Shore Drive at North Michigan Avenue, with some guest rooms with baths wide enough for wheelchair access.

All around winner for elegance, however, is the new **Ritz Carlton Hotel,** off North Michigan Avenue on Pearson Street, within the Water Tower Place complex. Of the 450 rooms, 30 were especially designed for the disabled. Whether you choose the Ritz as home while in Chicago or not, you'll want to discover its beautiful public rooms (see Day #1 itinerary for details).

Other hotels with special wheelchair facilities include:

Hyatt Regency Chicago, 151 East Wacker Drive
Marriott Motor Hotel, 8535 West Higgins
Holiday Inn–Lake Shore Drive, 644 North Lake Shore Drive.

Hotels claiming to be able to accommodate wheelchair travelers are:

Conrad Hilton, 720 South Michigan Avenue;
Palmer House, State and Monroe streets;
Pick Congress Hotel, 520 South Michigan Avenue;
Playboy Towers, 163 East Walton Street;
Sheraton-Chicago Hotel, 505 North Michigan Avenue.

Scheduled to open in 1978 is the new **Marriott Hotel** on North Michigan Avenue, a 1200-room hostelry with 20 rooms for the nonambulatory.

Although room rates are high in Chicago, you can take advantage of a variety of tour packages that range from $40 to $90 per person for two nights, including breakfasts and cocktails. For a list of the latest offerings, write to the Chicago Convention and Tourism Bureau or see your local travel agent.

## What You'll See and Do

With at least four days and a car at your disposal for one of these days, you'll see Chicago's art, history, and science museums; the best of her architecture and elegant shopping complexes; and sample her park with its zoo and conservatory. With a little more time, you'll enjoy the lake for a half day, venturing down a long walkway for a breath of fresh air or even fishing from a pier. And with more time you can explore her shops and museums thoroughly, drive outside the city to other destinations, and enjoy more of her restaurants and nighttime activities.

No matter what, take the time to discover elegant Chicago. In a morning or afternoon roll along North Michigan Avenue, perhaps stopping at the famous **Wally Findlay Gallery** for a look at the latest exhibit of original French impressionist paintings. Stop for a cup of tea or lunch at the chic **Jacques Garden** (one step) in the women's specialty shop called **Stanley Korshak.** Plan on dining in at least one of the great, glittering restaurants—perhaps the **Consort** in the Continental Plaza or **The Ninety-Fifth** at John Hancock Center.

But most important, don't forget to indulge in the city's rarest treasure, honest-to-goodness Chicago pizza-in-the-pan. A deep-dish pie of Sicilian origins, this version seems only to be available in Chicago. The best bet for a take-out order is **Pizzeria Uno's** at 29 East Ohio Street.

Other accessible restaurants in the North Michigan Avenue area include:

Adolph's, 1045 North Rush Street
Agostino's, 7 East Delaware Place
Atlantic Restaurant, 7115 West Grand Avenue
Blackhawk, 110 East Pearson Street
Bon Ton, 1153 North State Street
Bratislava, 2527 North Clark Street
Cape Cod Room, Drake Hotel, 140 East Walton Street (enter off North Michigan Avenue)

Consort, Continental Plaza Hotel, 909 North Michigan
Avenue

Cricket's, Tremont Hotel, 100 East Chestnut Street

Eli's, 215 East Chicago Avenue

The Greenhouse, Ritz Carlton Hotel, 160 East Pearson Street

Hugo's Gourmet Restaurant, Water Tower Hyatt House, 800
North Michigan Avenue

The Mezzanine Restaurants, Water Tower Place, 835 North
Michigan Avenue

Mushroom & Sons, 1 East Scott Street

The Ninety-Fifth, John Hancock Center, 175 East Delaware
Street

Ron of Japan, 230 East Ontario Street

Sherlock's Home, 900 North Michigan Avenue (enter from
Delaware Street)

The Terrace, Ritz Carlton Hotel, 160 East Pearson Street

Wrigley Restaurant, 410 North Michigan Avenue

For information on restaurants, cultural happenings and events
get a copy of *Key* or *Where* magazines in your hotel lobby. For another good resource, pick up a copy of the free *Reader*, a publication that comes out on Thursday nights in local stores. And for
those special questions relating to wheelchair travel, call *Rollin' On*
adviser Jack Catlin at the Rehabilitation Institute of Chicago,
(312) 649–6190.

## TOUR 1

WHAT YOU'LL DO

- Cab tour along Gold Coast, Lake Shore Drive.
- Self-tour of Lincoln Park Zoo and Conservatory.
- Lunch and shop at the Warehouse.
- Visit Chicago Historical Society.
- Cab tour of historic Astor Street.
- Self-tour of North Michigan Avenue, Water Tower Place.

$___/$___ indicates adult/child admission fees.
† All sites listed under "Restrooms" offer accessible facilities with wide
stall doors and grab bars unless otherwise indicated.

- Libations at the 96th-floor lounge of the John Hancock Building.
- Stop at Hugo's outdoor cafe.

HOW YOU'LL DO IT

- Cab from the hotel to Lincoln Park Zoo, 100 West Webster Street.
- Push three blocks to Warehouse complex, 1750 North Clark Street.
- Push from Warehouse to Chicago Historical Society, North Clark at West North Avenue, enter from Clark Street.
- Cab from Society via Astor Street to Saks Fifth Avenue or Water Tower Place; enter from garage off Pearson or Chestnut streets.
- Push within Water Tower Place, then to John Hancock Center across street at 835 North Michigan Avenue; enter from Chestnut Street.
- Push from Center to Hugo's outdoor cafe, Water Tower Hyatt Hotel, Chestnut at North Michigan Avenue.
- Push or cab from cafe to hotel.

THINGS TO KNOW

- Lincoln Park Zoo open 9:00 A.M.–5:00 P.M. daily, free admission.
- Rusty Scupper Restaurant in the Warehouse serves lunch from 1:30 to 2:30 P.M. daily.
- Chicago Historical Society open 9:00 A.M.–5:00 P.M. daily. Admission $1/50¢; free Mondays.
- Water Tower Place shops close at 6:00 or 7:00 P.M. on weekdays, but Mall open for window shopping, and several restaurants serve until 11:00 P.M. Sunday–Thursday, 'til 1:00 A.M. Friday and Saturday.
- John Hancock Center observatory open 9:00 A.M.–midnight. Admission $1.50/$1. The Ninety-Fifth Restaurant and 96th-floor Sybaris Lounge open 6:00 to 11:30 P.M.
- Hugo's at the Water Tower Hyatt Hotel open for lunch 11:30 A.M.–2:30 P.M., dinner 5:30–11:30 P.M.

RESTROOMS †

- Zoo (restroom accessible, but narrow stalls)
- Warehouse, ground floor (no grab bars)
- Chicago Historical Society
- Water Tower Place

Talk about elegance! As if seeing the Gold Coast and the Magnificent Mile weren't enough, today you'll also see a $3.3 million glass-enclosed house for apes complete with air conditioning, showers, and overhead sun lamps.

For eye openers, go by cab from your hotel to Lincoln Park following the famous Gold Coast portion of Lake Shore Drive. Once the residence of Chicago's business and social celebrities, this eight-block stretch of real estate fronting Lake Michigan is now the site for the city's most expensive apartments and condominiums. It's New York's Park Avenue with a lakefront view. As you pass the entranceways and lobbies you'll glimpse more crystal, mirrors, and sumptuous carpeting than inside the Hapsburg palaces of Austria. Highpoint of elegance is the Carlyle at 1040 North Lake Shore Drive, a delicately shaded green edifice with condominiums in the $100,000 to $200,000 price range.

Biggest star of the neighborhood, however, is Lake Michigan itself with its quiet blue water, waves crashing against stone seawalls, and sandy beaches tended by city lifeguards in snappy orange togs.

Lincoln Park stretches from the lake along almost the entire north end of the city. Focal point of this 1,185-acre reserve of old oak and hawthorn trees is the **Lincoln Park Zoo,** which came into being in 1868 when the city got two swans from New York's Central Park. Today the zoo rambles over 35 acres and houses 2600 animals, birds, and reptiles. Over four million people visit it each year, making it the most visited zoo in the country.

Among the highpoints are the fancy new ape house, which shelters the greatest collection of great apes in captivity, the country's finest man-made oasis for wild birds, a new sea lion pool with accessible underwater observation area, the zoo farm, and the children's zoo.

At the children's zoo just inside the main entrance, you'll see new-born and orphaned lions, tigers, jaguars, leopards, apes, and gorillas being hand raised in a nursery. You'll also watch children petting, hugging, and feeding the tame baby animals enclosed in a special garden.

By following the path that goes by the elephant enclosure, you'll come to the rock gardens of the **Lincoln Park Conservatory,** which adjoins the zoo. You can visit a portion of the main buildings to see the famous horticultural collection that includes an extensive orchid display. Spread in front of the buildings are formal gardens and a lovely fountain. Pass through these gardens toward the Schiller monument to return to the main entrance.

From the entrance you can roll to the zoo's Cafe Brauer, off the central mall overlooking the south pond, and enjoy a light lunch. Or, if you're left with a good supply of energy or assistance, you can wheel to the colorful Warehouse, with its restaurants and shops. If the Warehouse is your choice, roll out the Farm Zoo driveway west across Stockton Drive to Clark Street. You can cross Clark Street at the stoplight, but you'll face four curbs. Instead, if you like to move fast, you can cross in midstreet to the meridian, then continue across the busy street with nary a curb to climb.

A flutter of colorful banners marks the entrance to the **Warehouse,** an indoor shopping complex housed in what once was a moving and storage warehouse. You'll see the original hoisting apparatus now used for suspending a cargo of flower-filled pots in elaborate macrame hangers. A skylight adds warmth to the rustic wooden and brick walls and to the tile floors.

A full complement of boutiques fills the two levels connected by elevator. See the antique store, with its iron gate and forest of green plants and trees. At the Cafe Hennessy you can sample freshly baked breads and pastries, crêpes, and goulash. If you're lucky, they'll be handing out free samples of their famous marzipan confection. The **Rusty Scupper** restaurant, set in a courtyard of flowerpots and flickering lanterns, features a large salad bar to complement its menu of hot and cold entrees.

The Warehouse is on the edge of Old Town's main street, Wells Street, which runs parallel with North Clark. Only the most adventurous should attempt Old Town, however, for the streets are torn up, the uncut curbs are very high, and not many of the stores are accessible. A more rewarding venture would be to roll back across Clark Street to the east side skirting the park, and roll south three blocks (over four uncut curbs) to the **Chicago Historical Society.** Here a woman in a calico dress and bonnet dyes yarn and weaves on an 1820s loom as part of the museum's program of showing how the pioneers lived. Bringing history to life is a major goal of this avant garde museum, which was founded over 125 years ago. Twice its total collection was burned—once in the great Chicago fire—and rebuilt again.

Today the exhibits revolve around the famous Charles H. Gunther collection, which the Society purchased in 1920. A portion of the Civil War and Lincoln memorabilia from this collection is on view, including an entire Civil War prison and the bed that Lincoln died in. In the Lincoln gallery one sees a replica of the log cabin where he was born, the desk and chair he used when he studied law, his top hat, bedroom slippers, and spectacles.

Most popular, perhaps, is the museum's changing exhibits of costumes from their extensive collection of 12,000 hats, handkerchiefs, gowns, gloves, suits, shoes, uniforms, and umbrellas. One might see General Lafayette's dressing gown, Washington's inaugural suit, Sally Rand's fans, L.B.J.'s Stetson, or a Playboy bunny costume.

As you head from the museum to North Michigan Avenue, ask your cabbie to drive via **Astor Street** so you can see the rare assemblage of town houses designed by the greatest turn-of-the-century architects. The houses that line either side of the historical residential street make up a wonderland of turrets, gables, conical roofs, classical cornices, and gambrel roofs with dormers. Look for the red brick Archbishop residence facing Lincoln Park on North Avenue, typical of the Queen Anne period. The May House at 1443 Astor is Richardson Romanesque, with rusticated granite walls, broad bay, arched entrance, and square columns. The Charnley house at 1365 Adler was designated a Chicago landmark in 1972; it was designed by Adler and Sullivan in 1892, who at that time employed young Frank Lloyd Wright. If you've obtained your copy of *The Astor Street District* (see "Planning Your Trip" for details), you'll know which other famous residences to look for.

If you're ready for your ramble down North Michigan Avenue, ask your driver to let you out at **Saks Fifth Avenue** and roll two blocks along the flower-lined street to **Water Tower Place.** If not, ask to be let out at the ground level of the **Ritz Carlton Hotel** and take the elevators to the second-level atrium.

**Water Tower Place,** a $164 million multi-use urban complex, houses an eight-level atrium of shops and restaurants, a theater, four cinemas, 260 luxury condominiums, and the 450-room Ritz Carlton Hotel. You can see all except the condominiums by boarding the elevator in the hotel lobby on street level (off the garage parking) and getting off at the twelfth-floor main hotel lobby and the second-floor access to the atrium complex.

You'll probably blink and sigh a "wow" or two when you get your first glimpse of the Great Gatsby world of gleaming marble and glass that's been created in the atrium. A glass-enclosed elevator links the shops and restaurants in this unique vertical heaven of delicately shaded marble, terraced gardens, waterfalls, and trees. As you roll around, you'll come upon a roster of famous shops, including **Marshall Field, Lord & Taylor, Halston, Sassoon, Courrèges, F.A.O. Schwarz,** and **La Boite Musique,** devoted to music boxes in shapes you'd never believe: a squirrel, a model T car, a model of Chicago's Water Tower, a bride, a windmill, a hot air balloon.

For dinner you can choose between a **McDonald's,** a Belgian waffle shop, **D. B. Kaplan's** delicatessen, the **Plitt Ice Cream Parlour,** the **Theater Cafe, The Mezzanine restaurants** that include both The Pearson Room and The Courtyard.

**The Courtyard** is set up like an old Chicago street scene, with iron gates, brick walls, street lamps, flower boxes, and food stalls. You choose from smorgasbord, a delicatessen, soda fountain, pastry shop, soup, crêpe or hamburger stands, then dine at wooden tables, perhaps overlooking Seneca Park. From 4:30 to 9:30 P.M. there's usually musical entertainment.

Behind The Courtyard is the more formal **Pearson Room,** which recreates a residence of Old Chicago days with its Victorian sofas, potted palms, and gold lamp shades.

Other dinner possibilities await you in the **Ritz Carlton Hotel.** Whether you're dining there or not, do continue up by elevator to the main lobby, with its central fountain beneath a decorative skylight. To one side of the massive lobby is The Greenhouse, a glass-walled cocktail area with Italian mosaic floors, walls of bamboo and lush overhanging vines. Opposite it is **The Cafe** for informal dining, and around the corner **The Terrace,** a more formal dining spot that features a landscaped garden.

You can glimpse these lovely restaurants as you follow the hotel's 120-foot-long promenade lined with glass cases displaying goods from around the world.

The ninety-fourth-floor observation lounge of the **Hancock Tower** will give you an eagle's eye view of what you've seen and will see in Chicago. So will the ninety-sixth-floor **Sybaris Lounge,** where you'll also enjoy some heady luxury, drink in hand. You can rationalize your choice nicely when you add up the difference between the $1.50 charge to get into the observatory and the price of a drink.

Either choice, you'll enter the building from Chestnut Street and look for a security guard or elevator operator to direct you to the elevators serving **The Ninety-Fifth Restaurant.** If you've chosen the **Sybaris Lounge** viewpoint, then the elevator will take you directly; otherwise the operator can take you down to the concourse level, from where you'll take a second elevator to the observatory—after you pay the admission. (This second elevator, which goes from the concourse to the observatory, can otherwise be reached only by escalator.) As you ascend skyward you can entertain yourself with thoughts of how the people living in the condominiums that make up this vertical city kid about the whitecaps in their bathtubs when the structure sways, which it does slightly during high east winds.

Surveying the city from your quarter-mile-high perch you'll see why Chicago is considered America's greenest and grassiest big metropolis. Fringes of trees line the riverfront and polka-dot the city. Water makes up a major part of the scene, not just the lake, but also the Chicago River with its many tributaries and a surprising number of lagoons, in addition to the blue swimming pools on top of many of the apartment houses along Lake Shore Drive.

On a clear day you'll see the bordering states of Wisconsin, Indiana, and Michigan, an ever-changing panorama of cargo ships and sailboats on the river, and a jigsaw puzzle of buildings.

If you've planned things right, you'll be sitting on top of the world at twilight to watch the lights speckling buildings that look like black lucite boxes, rising like a thermometer along the sides of other structures, floodlighting the ornate roofs of still others.

Of course it will be hard to miss seeing the world's tallest building, **Sears Tower,** or "Big Buck" as the locals call this 110-story mammoth. Spectacular, too, are the white marble-sheathed Standard Oil Building, the undulating glass towers of Lakepoint Towers, the cylindrical Marina City.

The Hancock Tower, with its distinctive solid crown of lights on its upper stories, can be appreciated best from the sky deck at Sears Tower or from the water's edge—such buildings need distance.

One that doesn't is the Gothic limestone Water Tower, one of the few surviving structures of the Great Chicago Fire. As you wheel from the Hancock Center to your hotel you'll probably pass this turreted, towered medieval castle that became a historical landmark in 1971. To appreciate it fully, you may want to stop at the outdoor cafe at the corner of North Michigan and Chestnut streets. From this vantage, you'll see in one long look Chicago's oldest and newest innovative architecture: In the foreground, the century-old Water Tower and in the background the future of America's cities as embodied in the Water Tower Place and the John Hancock Center.

## TOUR 2

WHAT YOU'LL DO

- View the city from the Navy Pier.
- Stop in the Olive Park garden of fountains.
* • Brunch at the Pinnacle Restaurant for a revolving view.
* • Explore the Field Museum of Natural History.
- Visit the Shedd Aquarium.
- Dine in or near your hotel.

* Indicates restriction in time of visit.
$___/$___ indicates adult/child admission fees.
† All sites listed under "Restrooms" offer accessible facilities with wide stall doors and grab bars unless otherwise indicated.

HOW YOU'LL DO IT

- Cab from your hotel to the Navy Pier, Streeter Drive at Illinois Avenue.
- Push from the Pier via Olive Park to the Holiday Inn—Lake Shore Drive at Ontario Street.
- Cab from the Holiday Inn to the Field Museum, Lake Shore Drive at Roosevelt Road. Use ramp to left of main entrance.
- Push with assistance through the underground ramped tunnel to Shedd Aquarium, Lake Shore Drive.
- Cab from Shedd Aquarium to hotel.
- Push into or from hotel to dinner.

THINGS TO KNOW

\* • Reservations necessary for Sunday brunch at the Pinnacle Restaurant.
\* • Field Museum open 9:00 A.M.–5:00 P.M. Admission $1.50/ 50¢. Weekend Discovery tours 11:00 A.M.–3:00 P.M.
- Shedd Aquarium open 9:00 A.M.–5:00 P.M. Admission $1.50/50¢. Films usually at 11:00 A.M. and 2:00 P.M., but best to check.

RESTROOMS †

- Navy Pier
- Holiday Inn–Lake Shore Drive
- Field Museum, ground floor
- Shedd Aquarium, mezzanine

A day for superlatives—a spectacular view of the city from the water's edge and then from a revolving restaurant while sipping champagne. Later you'll see the world's greatest museum of natural history and then the largest collection of fish anywhere.

To conclude such a spectacular day appropriately is not easy, but it is possible. By dining at one of Chicago's sumptuous restaurants you'll come close.

Begin with a cab ride to the entrance to the **Navy Pier.** You can roll along this arm that juts 3000 feet into the lake, going a quarter mile or so to the tip with its half dome shell where concerts are held. If you don't want to go that far, stop a few feet down the walkway for a look at the city and the passing boats and to find out if the fishermen are catching anything.

Just 100 yards south of the entrance to the Navy Pier stands an unlikely gourmet haven, **Rocky & Sons,** a bait shop so famous for its deep-fried shrimp that bicyclists, joggers, wheelers, and in-the-know Chicagoans keep it a secret. You can find out what all the fuss is about by wheeling over the rough road, buying a portion, and nibbling it at water's edge.

Should your taste have higher sights, head for the Holiday Inn across the street, with its revolving **Pinnacle Restaurant** on top. Your route will take you through Olive Park, actually a water filtration center that's been beautifully disguised. While enjoying Sunday brunch, including complimentary champagne, you'll see what may be the most spectacular view in town.

From the Holiday Inn it's a short cab ride to the **Field Museum of Natural History,** one of the world's greatest repositories. In 1976 the Museum opened a new ground-level public entrance for the disabled as part of a $25 million renovation program. It has a ramped access on the west side of the building.

Scientist and humanitarian Jacob Bronowski spoke of "the fierce elation that accompanies man's endless quest to know himself and his environment." Something of that fierce elation can be experienced when you enter the dimly lit Hall of Dinosaurs at the Field Museum of Natural History and sense the world of 150 million years ago. Clues, insights, and revelations of the distant past abound in this place of discovery, thanks to a staff alive with ideas on how to present the collection. Every modern exhibit device is used, from diorama and life-sized figures to exhibit films and environmental scenes.

Exemplifying this sophisticated ability to exhibit the collection in relevant settings is the new "Man in His Environment" exhibit. In six distinct areas the exhibit integrates anthropology, botany, and zoology to dramatize the meaning of ecology. By using environments, diorama, and film, this exhibit illustrates earth's diversity, the working of natural laws, the increasing complexity of food-producing tools, and then shows how other cultures have lived harmoniously with their environment. A film in "The Choice Is Ours" portion of the exhibit presents the status and alternatives for growth, encouraging visitors to consider the implications for man's future.

To help the visitor get an overview of the total museum collection that is exhibited in the forty-eight exhibit halls and galleries, the main floor Anniversary Exhibit presents stunning examples from each of the four scientific disciplines that the museum encompasses. Another good way to see some of the Museum highlights or special exhibits is by joining the Weekend Discovery tour conducted by volunteer docents.

What if you want to see the highlights of the total collection? Then you can choose from among these show-stoppers:

- The best preserved ancient ship in existence: an Egyptian funerary vessel
- Some of the most important native American art objects in the country: a Pawnee drum and ghost dance dress
- The only free-standing dinosaur skeleton in the United States
- The finest examples of taxidermy in the world: two fighting bull elephants
- African Water Hole, an outstanding example of animals mounted in their natural environment
- Hopewell Indian exhibit, especially the ornaments
- Painted buffalo robe that almost certainly belonged to Chief Joseph of the Nez Percé
- Probably the country's finest example of Plains Indians' realistic art: two Cheyenne buffalo robes covered with hand-painted depictions of war exploits
- Dioramas showing aspects of Aztec and Mayan civilizations in exquisite detail
- Hall of Gems
- Skeleton of a brontosaurus
- Life-size statues depicting mankind around the world
- Exceptionally fine examples of marine mammals, collected on Admiral Richard E. Byrd's second Antarctic expedition

Whether you see the high points, join a tour, or head for your favorite kind of collection, be sure to take a tea break in the charming museum cafe, and look into the museum shop with its African baskets and Indian jewelry.

When you're ready, leave by the door you came in and use the 100-foot-long ramp that goes under Lake Shore Drive to reach the Shedd Aquarium. (You'll need assistance because the ramp is steep.) At the north entrance to the left you'll find a ramp that connects with the education department elevator. Generally there's someone around to run the elevator, but if not you can ask someone to call an attendant for you; if you want to be sure, call the Aquarium before leaving the Field Museum and let them know you're on your way.

Seeing the underwater life in the **Shedd Aquarium**'s new coral reef tank is like snorkeling 12 feet into the reefs of the Caribbean. The 6-foot high windows of the 125-foot circular glass tank bring you into a world where 6-foot eels lurk, neon goby dart, barracudas cruise, and lazy nurse sharks rest. You are eyeball to eyeball with sawfish, sharks, and skates and almost seventy-five other kinds of denizens.

This coral reef of simulated vase sponges, mauve-colored sea whips, white brain coral and lacy sea fans is so realistic that the fish don't seem to know the difference. In fact the fish are so at home in their pseudoworld of rubber and plastic coral that some drive off opponents that try to invade it and nibble at it, as they do in nature. One fish, the parrotfish, intent on munching the phony polyp growth inspired the curator to install polyp of a more edible nature—plaster of paris mixed with tuna fish.

As this cast of about one thousand fish darts, dives, and dances on its underwater stage, lights, music, and sound narration turn the show into a major production. A fully automated lighting system suspended over the tank provides a programmed sequence of effects from full daylight to sundown and night. Interspersed with these dusk-to-night effects are spotlights dramatizing parts of the reef or particular types of coral. Musical scores like the 101 Strings rendering "Ebb Tide" or Les Baxter's orchestra striking up "Tahiti: A Summer Night at Sea" do their part to sweep you away. A narrator brings you back to reality with information about the intricate interrelationship of living organisms you see and their place in a total ecological system.

Twice a day a diver with a bucket of food descends to dispense squirts of brine shrimp or foot-long mackerels. Using a mask microphone, the diver lets viewers in on his communications with the fish. One of the most popular repartees is the one between the diver and Mort the eel, who has to be coaxed to eat his mackerel supper instead of biting into "a nice leg."

The special films shown in the Aquarium theater on weekends tell how the Aquarium crew captures its specimens. The free movies are shown at 11:00 A.M. and 2:00 P.M. on most Saturdays and Sundays, but it's best to check exact times as soon as you arrive.

Although the movies and fascinating coral reef display can take up most of your time, you may want to put aside at least a few minutes to marvel at the Russian sturgeon. The fish came to the Aquarium in 1971 as a 4-inch specimen and today is one of the largest fish in captivity—seven amazing feet! Another eye-catcher is the freshwater dolphin from the Amazon River. With more time you can see others of the six galleries displaying 5400 different kinds of fish—the largest collection in the world.

If the little hand on the enchanting fish clock has not reached the squid (5:00 o'clock) when you're done with your tour, visit the special Sea Shop, where you'll find an extensive collection of shells and such unusual items as shark jaws, sea urchin lamps, and a battery-operated wave machine.

You can return to your hotel via Lake Shore Drive if you would like to enjoy the lake again. For dinner choose among the restaurants in your hotel or nearby. Perhaps this will be the night for that sumptuous dinner, so you can experience Chicago elegance with all your senses.

## TOUR 3

WHAT YOU'LL DO

- Shop, sightsee, and lunch at Marshall Field.
- Tour the Loop by cab for a look at the Chagall mosaic, Picasso sculpture, and Calder sculpture, with optional stop at Sears Tower for skydeck view.

* Indicates restriction in time of visit.
$___/$___ indicates adult/child admission fees.
† All sites listed under "Restrooms" offer accessible facilities with wide stall doors and grab bars unless otherwise indicated.

* • Visit to Art Institute, with dinner in museum cafe (open Thursday nights).
• Attend evening performance at Orchestra Hall.

### HOW YOU'LL DO IT

• Cab from your hotel to Marshall Field & Company, 111 North State Street.
• Cab tour of the Loop, then to the Art Institute, Michigan Avenue at Adams Street. Use 125 East Monroe Street entrance.
• Conducted tour and self-tour of Art Institute.
• Push across the street to Orchestra Hall, 220 South Michigan Avenue.
• Cab from Orchestra Hall to hotel.

### THINGS TO KNOW

• Marshall Field opens at 10:00 A.M. There are five restaurants on the seventh floor and an ice cream parlor on the third floor.
* • Art Institute open 10:30 A.M.–8:00 P.M. Thursday; 10:30–4:30 P.M. Monday–Friday; from 10:00 A.M.–5:00 P.M. Saturday; noon to 5:00 P.M. Sunday. Suggested voluntary donation $2/$1. Thursdays free. One-hour lectures Sunday at 3:15 P.M., Thursday at 6:15 P.M.
• Orchestra Hall is the home of the famed Chicago Symphony Orchestra. Reserve tickets (see Planning Your Trip for details).

### RESTROOMS †

• Art Institute
• Marshall Field & Co. (standard stall 24 inches wide)

Today you'll find out why Chicago is called "the city that does things big." After you're most likely dazzled by a 6000-foot Tiffany dome, puzzled by Picasso and Calder sculptures, and have admired Chagall's stained glass windows, you'll see a collection of French impressionist paintings that may rival those in the Louvre.

Begin with a cab ride to the world-famous **Marshall Field De-**

**partment Store.** Ask your cab driver to approach it via Madison Street so you can see Louis Sullivan's greatest masterpiece, the **Carson Pirie Scott Building.** Note the delicately detailed cast iron ornamentation on the first two floors.

At Marshall Field, head for the glove department, a good place to view the fabulous dome of 1,600,000 pieces of glass built under the direction of Louis C. Tiffany.

Explore the store as interest directs you, but don't miss the Trend House on the eighth floor, which is redecorated each year to spotlight a special period. On the third floor you'll find a turn-of-the-century ice cream parlour and for more serious lunching **The Heather House** on the eighth floor. On the seventh floor, **five restaurants** circle a promenade that opens onto a huge light well. Here you can make your own sandwich, enjoy a full hot meal for a set price, lunch in a cafeteria that looks like grandma's kitchen or luxuriate in a pretty room with flower-bordered fountain as centerpiece.

When you're ready to go, settle back in your cab for a brief tour of several of the city's contemporary art forms. See the 50-foot-high rusty steel sculpture at the Civic Center by Picasso, "The Four Seasons" mosaic by Marc Chagall at the First National Bank Plaza, and the indefinable "Scarlet Flamingo" by Alexander Calder at Federal Center.

At the **Art Institute of Chicago** get out at the Monroe Street entrance, where you'll experience wheeler's nirvana. One wheeler said of the beautiful plaza and gardens at the rear of the Institute: "It's better than the entrance in front of the building! It's the best I've ever seen." The new plaza and gardens are part of the Institute's new wing, which is a model of accessibility. The free-standing archway dominating the garden is the main entrance from the famous Chicago New York Stock Exchange Building, which has been reconstructed and restored inside the Institute's new wing. You can see the room with its colored glass skylight, cast-plaster ornamentation, intricate stenciled ceiling, Honduras mahogany paneling, and red oak floors.

Also part of this new wing is the elegant **Members' Lounge,** open to the public from 11:00 A.M. to 2:30 P.M., a cafeteria, and a garden cafe, open only when the sun shines. As you begin your tour you'll pass the new Marc Chagall "American Windows," unveiled in 1977. In six 8-foot-high glass panels, the artist celebrates America, as lovers, dancers, and animals float, dance, and spin with flowers, moons, and stars above a Chicago cityscape.

Beyond McKinlock Court with its fringe of old elm trees lies the main part of the building exhibits, a permanent collection of Oriental art and French and post-impressionist paintings. The impressionist collection, with its paintings by Van Gogh, Toulouse-Lautrec, Renoir, Seurat, and Monet, is believed by many to outrank that of the Louvre. To make sure you don't miss the most important pieces, pick up the Institute's booklet *Not to Be Missed,* which tells you where to find the top twelve masterpieces.

As you roll through the spacious galleries, be sure to include a stop to see the "Thorne Rooms in Miniature" exhibit. These miniature period rooms, first shown at the 1939 Golden Gate Exposition in San Francisco, are faithful copies of famous rooms in historic landmarks and museums around the world. Since no museum can hope to provide the public with a complete series of fully furnished period rooms, these miniature versions give a rare perspective of the world of interior decor.

If you've planned your visit as suggested for a Thursday evening, you can dine in the cheerful museum cafeteria and then attend the one-hour free lecture given at 6:15 P.M. Following the lecture and a visit to the extensive museum shop, it will be time to proceed to **Orchestra Hall** across the street.

If you've obtained tickets for a performance of the Chicago Symphony Orchestra, your day that opened with a Tiffany dome will close fittingly with music played by one of the world's most famous orchestras.

## TOUR 4

WHAT YOU'LL DO

- Visit the Museum of Science and Industry, with lunch in the Museum Cafe.

† All sites listed under "Restrooms" offer accessible facilities with wide stall doors and grab bars unless otherwise indicated.

HOW YOU'LL DO IT

- Drive eight miles south to the Museum, 57th Street and Lake Shore Drive. Use ramped north entrance.

THINGS TO KNOW

- Museum open 9:30 A.M.–5:30 P.M. daily except on weekdays in the Labor Day thru April period, when the Museum closes at 4:00 P.M. Admission is free. Cafeteria open to public and also Finnigan's Ice Cream Parlor open 11:30 A.M.–3:30 P.M. weekdays, 11:00 A.M.–5:00 P.M. weekends.

RESTROOMS †

- Museum of Science and Industry

One of the main reasons most tourists come to Chicago in the first place is so they can play like kids again, pushing, pressing, turning, cranking and pulling buttons, cranks, levers, and wheels at the **Museum of Science and Industry.** Even if you don't think you like science this museum that shows you how principles of science are applied in industry and everyday life will captivate you.

Plan on spending all day, seeing and doing as much as you can. Your day will be filled with such experiences as being guided by a miner wearing a hard hat and electric lamp into a coal mine. You'll ride the hoist (elevator) that lowers passengers into the heart of the mine shaft. You'll smell the dank coal diggings, hear the clatter of giant machines, and see real southern Illinois coal in tunnels.

You'll also go to a circus via a ramp that passes miniature figures bringing the three ring Big Top to life. At the new "Food for Life" exhibit you'll see an open-air marketplace with stalls of wax-and-vinyl fruits and vegetables, watch hatching chicks, and participate in the testing of food products. At "Yesterday's Main Street" exhibit you'll roll down cobblestoned, gas-lit streets of 1910 to old Finnigan's Pharmacy, now serving twentieth-century ice cream sodas and banana splits.

Not to be missed is the famous Colleen Moore Fairy Castle, now in its own room complete with organ music background. In the dollhouse castle you'll see running water, a dinner service made by Royal Doulton, an alabaster and gold bathroom with a bearskin rug made from ermine with tiny mouse teeth sewn in, and a weeping willow that weeps watery tears.

In the seventy-five exhibit halls that cover fourteen acres you'll see everything from a car of the future and a Santa Fe model railway to a typical hospital operating room and a 16-foot walkthrough heart.

A visit to the Museum plus a refreshing drive along Lake Shore Drive nicely concludes a visit to Chicago. Both are hard acts to follow:

## Other Accessible Attractions

Academy of Science
Adler Planetarium
Chicago Fire Academy
Chicago Public Library
Chicago Stadium
Chicago Sun-Times Daily News
Chicago Tribune
Chicago Mercantile Exchange
McCormick Place-on-the-Lake
Piper Alley
Quaker Oats Kitchens
Sears Tower
Soldier Field
Wrigley Field

INTRODUCING
*Rollin' On* adviser, wheeler Jack Catlin

*Title*: Director ACCESS Chicago, Rehabilitation Institute
*Telephone number*: (312) 649–6190
*Hometown*: Chicago
*Favorite tourist site*: Chagall windows at the Art Institute
*Hidden corner*: Rusty Scupper restaurant at the Warehouse
*Rendezvous*: The Greenhouse at the Ritz Carlton Hotel
*Offbeat restaurant*: Diana's Grocery Store and Restaurant, 1305
     Halstead Street (Greek)

*Place for Music*: the Navy Pier, Grant Park, or Amazing Grace in Evanston

*View*: from top of Sears Tower

*Natural wonder*: Lake Michigan

*Museum*: Museum of Science and Industry

*Ramble*: from Lincoln Park Zoo over the south pedestrian over-pass over Lake Shore Drive to the walkway skirting the lake

*Non-tourist destination*: the fishing platform at Olive Park, a water filtration plant overlooking the lake

*Offbeat experience*: fishing in the Lincoln Park lagoons

*Traditional restaurant*: Mushroom & Sons

*Low-cost restaurant*: steak and eggs at Mitchell's Restaurant, 1201 North State Street

*Ice cream shop*: Baskin-Robbins, 505 North Michigan

*Reading suggestion*: *Boss* by Mike Royko

*Place to get a wheelchair repaired*: Aamed Inc., Forrest Park

*Tip on having a great time in Chicago*: Hear music at the Bandshell during the summer, try Chicago pizza at Uno's, go to Water Tower Place for beautiful shops and smiles.

# 6

# Honolulu

Waving palms, white sand beaches, tropical flowers, sweet, smiling people—the classic words of description that float to the mind at the mention of Hawaii. But they're only words, gestures at describing an honest-to-goodness paradise that must be experienced to be believed.

Such experiencing can happen anytime: when the sea turns luminous blue and the white sand glows pink at sunset, when the breeze touches your brow like the hand of a dear friend, when the fragrance of ginger comes to haunt you. Your senses turn on as never before. You know at once that you've never really seen color before this moment, nor felt the breeze, nor smelled a flower.

That's one side of paradise for sure. Another is the people of the islands, especially the native Hawaiians, who look as if they have some wonderful secret about happiness they may share at any moment. Instead they smile and joke with you, laughing whenever they can, and if it's not appropriate to laugh they sing.

These cheerful Hawaiians, who somehow always have time to be helpful, go a long way toward making any wheelchair traveler's visit to the Islands a delight. As an islander wheeler sums it up, "We're long on helping people." What that means is that in Honolulu the wheelchair traveler can go places and do things he or she might not be able to do elsewhere.

For instance, the beach boys on Waikiki Beach will assist you or even carry you, if you'd like, to sit at the water's edge or so that you can ride a canoe or catamaran. Paved walkways, narrow but negotiable, link many hotels with the beach. You wheel to where the walkway ends, ask someone to get a beach boy for you, or make arrangements ahead of time through your hotel for one to meet you.

That same willingness to do special things for people has something to do with the existence of Handi-Cab, America's only wheel-aboard taxicab fleet. This twenty-four hour cab service includes the assistance of a carefully trained driver who knows how to handle a wheelchair and will cheerfully get you up, around, and into just about any place you want to go. Such service opens up the restaurant and nightclub scene to wheelers; you can go to any show without getting out of your chair and know that when the show is over you'll be picked up.

Many of the boat cruises also become possible when there are people on hand to assist you aboard. A moonlight dinner cruise, a watery tour to Pearl Harbor, a sail on a catamaran—all become things wheelchair travelers can do in Hawaii. Honolulu advisor Lowell Grant recommends the free Navy boat that goes out of Halaway gate of Pearl Harbor to the *Arizona* Memorial; they're "more than happy to help handicapped people aboard."

Best of all, Waikiki Beach is a place you can get around nicely by yourself. The wide, flat main street that skirts the ocean is totally curb ramped. You could spend your entire vacation just rolling around Waikiki, stopping under a banyan tree beside the sea, watching the shows at a dozen hotels, catching the free entertainment on the street and in hotel lobbies, shopping at the fascinating International Market, eating and sipping in dozens of restaurants and nightclubs.

The quality and quantity of entertainment available in Waikiki may surprise you. Of course, there's enough Hawaiian song and dance to satisfy anyone, but there's also much more: piano bars, comics, modern musical reviews, and jazz groups. During the cocktail hours, many hotels put on free entertainment in their lobbies, and others in their cocktail terraces—where for the price of a drink you can see some of the best Hawaiian entertainers around. But after the sun sets you can see some of the most lavish productions this side of Las Vegas in the showrooms around Waikiki. Among the choices: a Polynesian aquacade that combines dinner with a

Hawaiian revue that's part hula, part fire dance, and part Ziegfeld Follies; a revue that features over thirty Tahitian, Samoan, Fijian, Maori performers (including fire dancers); an evening of authentic chants, hulas, songs, and costumes from the monarchy period; Chinese cuisine followed by precision acrobats, magicians, and Kung Fu opera.

In addition to the lively entertainment to be found in the Waikiki hotels and clubs, Hawaii has its share of cultural events. The modern Blaisdell Center, a complex of entertainment and convention facilities, is the site for a number of musical events, including performances by the Hawaii Opera Theater and Honolulu Symphony Orchestra. For theater the Honolulu Community Theatre, Hawaii Performing Arts Company, University of Hawaii Theatre, and other groups present Broadway hits and classics. A number of free concerts are also staged at the Waikiki Shell, an open-air concert hall in the Kapiolani Park. All are accessible.

## Planning Your Trip

Anytime's a good time to go to Hawaii. Temperatures in the subtropical islands average 75 degrees year around. There can be some humid days in August and some rainy ones between November and March, but humid days and rainy days are interspersed with mild sunny ones year 'round. During the summer there's lots going on, including free concerts, but the summer rates usually are higher at hotels, and restaurants are crowded. All things considered, spring, fall and early winter are top choices, with Aloha Week in mid-October coming in as top contender. During this eight-day-long celebration you'll have the bonus of seeing everything from an orchid show to dance events and demonstrations of ancient arts and crafts.

Literature about Aloha Week, about the tourist attractions, hotels—everything—can be obtained by writing to the Hawaii Visitors Bureau at 2270 Kalakaua Avenue, Honolulu, Hawaii 96815, or by contacting one of the branch offices in Los Angeles, San Francisco, Chicago, or New York.

One thing you won't want to miss doing while in Hawaii is attending a luau. If you have a friend or associate who, in advance, can consult the local newspapers for a listing of one given at a church or by a civic group, great. Otherwise begin looking through the papers when you arrive and try to plan on attending. You'll find those given by private groups to be friendly, lively, and delicious. If you can't go to a private luau, however, try those given by hotels. You'll find information on them listed in the tourist newspapers and magazines available on the street or in the hotel lobby.

If you'll have some time in Honolulu, you may want to make a note to contact the Easter Seal Society there to learn about the upcoming activities of the Adult Recreation Center for the Handicapped (ARCH). ARCH puts on periodic bowling meets, picnics, trips, and potluck suppers; guests are always welcome.

Should you have a special problem or question, or want to have your wheelchair repaired, call on *Rollin' On* adviser Lowell Grant at (808) 533-2794. Lowell knows just about anything you can think to ask about Hawaii. He'll also rent and install a hand-controlled device on your rental car.

### Getting There

Only in Hawaii would you find an airport with a garden island filled with tropical blooms and circled by white swans. In fact the airport is embellished by three tropical gardens: one Japanese style, another Chinese, and the third Hawaiian. You'll probably catch sight of one as you roll from your arriving airplane, but if not, plan on getting to the airport a little early for your return trip so you'll have a few minutes to enjoy this unusual airport amenity.

The modern Honolulu International Airport also offers wheelchair-accessible facilities, including restrooms and restaurant. Located about nine miles from Waikiki, the taxi cab transfer is a short pleasant trip and costs about $8.

### Getting Around

Handi-Cab, a wheel-aboard van that operates like a taxicab, makes an ideal form of transportation, especially for getting around Waikiki Beach in the evenings. You can remain in your chair and know that you'll be picked up on schedule when the nightclub show concludes or whenever you say or call. The rates are $3 per pickup and 80¢ per mile, but the van with driver can also be rented for $14 per hour. Renting the van at $14 an hour particularly makes sense when you're traveling with several friends. They need not all be disabled, as the van accommodates four people in chairs and four who are ambulatory. A tour around the island, for instance, which takes about eight hours, costs $112 for one person or $14 for each of eight people. With this in mind, it's a good idea to call Handi-Cab as soon as you arrive, letting them know you'd like to get together with other chair travelers who are renting a van and don't have the maximum number of people to fill the van. Then if a tour comes up, you'll be called and can decide if the destination and timing suit you.

In addition to the taxicab rate and the hourly rate, Handi-Cab also offers another option. It's a moonlight dinner cruise aboard a catamaran for $19.50 that includes roundtrip van transportation to and from your hotel. A second package offers a daytime cruise to Pearl Harbor for $9, including transportation.

Perhaps nowhere else do you have as many opportunities for being on the water than in Hawaii. In addition to the Handi-Cab cruise package, you can take a number of other cruises and even go by jet hydrofoil to any of the neighboring islands except Lanai. The hydrofoils are all accessible and many of the other cruise boats are also. When you make a reservation you can inquire about boarding procedures.

Although most of Hawaii's main tourist attractions are within a few miles of Waikiki and can be done by Handi-Cab or conventional taxicab, you probably will want to rent a car for at least one day so you can visit other parts of the island.

Presently Avis is the only car rental company offering hand-controlled automobiles in the Islands. By ordering your vehicle ahead (see Chapter 2 for details) you should have no problem. But as an alternative, keep Lowell Grant's phone number handy; he's the wheeler who repairs chairs and rents hand control devices. He'll actually come down to the car rental agency to meet you and install a device on the spot (his phone number is in the Planning Your Trip portion of this chapter).

Conventional taxicabs are plentiful even if you do occasionally have to wait while the driver finishes an animated conversation with a hotel bellman. Once inside the cab, you run the risk of finding a new lifelong friend, for if the driver likes you, he'll give you his card and from then on you have your own personal driver—and an amusing tour guide for your time in the Islands.

If you're not being transported by land or by sea, you have another delightful option in Waikiki, pushing yourself down the wide, flat, totally curb-ramped main street that follows the curve of the ocean for about two miles. If you were to go no place else on Oahu but up and down Kalakaua Avenue, you could, as many tourists do, amuse yourself for days with the fascinating string of shops, restaurants, and hotels, not to mention the beachside walkways overlooking the sea and the shady arbors and poolside terraces at almost every hotel.

They say that Waikiki is like that cafe in Paris. If you sit under the palms beside the beach long enough, you'll meet everyone in the world you've ever known. That's one of the great things about paradise—sometimes you can just sit pretty and wait for the world to come to you.

## Where to Stay

Since Waikiki is such a wonderland of curb ramps and accessibility, it's where you want to be. Besides, the beach area is where the action is. Whether you stay at a beachfront hotel with its own plot of sand or not, you still can enjoy the beach scene, since the lovely Kuhio Beach Park beside the Moana Hotel is public land. It also happens to be one of the best natural beaches in Waikiki, with a walkway that juts out into the water and shady arbors along the street, where you can sit and watch the bikini-dotted sand.

Exactly where you'll stay along Waikiki Beach will have a great deal to do with what you want to see and particularly how you like to spend your evenings. At the Ewa end of Waikiki, you can stay at the accessible **Ilikai,** 1777 Ala Moana Avenue, a world within itself with great restaurants, entertainment, miles of outdoor walkways, patios, terraces, pools—the works.

The **Sheraton Waikiki,** 2255 Kalakaua Avenue, is just as much a world in itself, somewhat separated from the street scene by the bordering gardens.

For the wheeler who wants to ramble on his own in the surf pounding heart of Waikiki—in the action center—your choice of accessible hotels includes the **Holiday Inn** or the **Hawaiian Regent.**

The 636-room **Holiday Inn–Waikiki Beach,** 2570 Kalakaua Avenue, is one of the most spacious and charming of the Holiday Inn chain. Best of all, it's situated just across the street from Kuhio Beach. Elevators connect the ground-floor entrance with the second-floor lobby, which opens onto a pool and terrace. Music begins here in the late afternoon, usually featuring a lively Hawaiian group, and continues into the evening. There are a number of restaurants. The Catamaran Lounge features entertainment from Polynesian music and dancing to contemporary rock.

The 690-room, twenty-five story **Hawaiian Regent Hotel,** 2552 Kalakaua Avenue, is one of Honolulu's newest. The outstanding feature of this hotel is its lush garden court complete with rippling stream. Some rooms, the lobby, and the public rooms open onto this open-air area with quiet corners for listening to the music that emanates from the Garden Court Lounge. Facilities include a terrace for swimming and sunning, three restaurants, a snack shop, nightclub, and the garden lounge.

If you're renting a car for your stay, the **Ala Moana Americana,** adjacent to the Ala Moana Shopping Center at 410 Atkinson Drive, would be a good choice. The hotel is completely accessible, it's central (although not on the beach), and one of the best big hotel bargains.

Although not currently offering rooms that are specifically designed for wheelchair travelers, the following hotels are accessible and are considered good bets by the people who put out the *Aloha Guide to Honolulu for the Handicapped*:

> Waikikian Hotel, 1811 Ala Moana Avenue
> Kahala Hilton, 5000 Kahala Avenue
> Waikiki Beachcomber, 2300 Kalakaua Avenue
> Cinerama Reef Hotel, 2169 Kala Road.

If you want to explore other possibilities among the 75 Waikiki hotels, you could refer to the *Hawaii Visitors Bureau Hotel Guide*, which is keyed for wheelchair accessibility. The accessibility, however, is loosely defined by the hotel owners themselves and requires additional inquiry by letter (see Chapter 2 hotel section for more details).

## What You'll See and Do

You'd think looking at the water, feeling the breeze, smelling the flowers, and eating fresh pineapple would be enough. Actually it is, but there's more if you want it—lots of superb sightseeing within a few miles of Waikiki. You can go by Handi-Cab or by conventional taxicab and see a jungle park filled with the world's most exotic birds, a recreation of a South Seas village, a handsomely renovated sugar mill, an oceanarium of performing dolphins, an ethnic corner that shows you a China to be seen nowhere else outside the Orient.

But with all these things to see and do, sightseeing still cannot be taken too seriously. So instead of day-long itineraries, a smattering of minitours (as well as one full-day tour) are offered here that can be combined for full day outings as your heart, sunshine, and soft breezes dictate. The minitours can be done by cab, but the day-long round-the-island tour requires a rented car, a friend with a car, or a Handi-Cab group.

A big part of any vacation in the Islands is the fun of sampling the wide variety of ethnic cuisines and eating in different ways, like at a luau, hukilau, or munching around the International Market Place. With this in mind, a list of restaurants known to be accessible is included so you can pick and choose as mood dictates.

### *Among the Accessible Restaurants*

American

> Bobby McGee's Conglomeration, Colony East Hotel, 2885
>     Kalakaua Avenue
> Canoe House, Ilikai Hotel, 1777 Ala Moana Boulevard
> Chuck's Steak House, Edgewater Hotel, 2168 Kalia Road

The Pottery Steak House, 3574 Waialae Avenue
Prince Kuhio's, Ala Moana Center
Tiki Broiler, International Market Place
Whalers Broiler, Ala Moana Americana
Willows, 901 Hausten Street
Victoria Station, Ala Moana Hotel

Chinese

Golden Dragon, Hilton Hawaiian Village
Mongolian Barbecue, Cultural Plaza, 100 North Beretania
Winter Garden, Kahala Mall
Wo Fat, 115 North Hotel Street (downstairs only)
Yangtze, Cultural Plaza, 100 North Beretania

Continental

Cafe Colonnade, Princess Kaiulani Hotel
Catamaran Restaurant, Holiday Inn–Waikiki
Canlis, 2100 Kalakaua Avenue
Cavalier, 1630 Kapiolani Boulevard
Hanohano Room, Sheraton–Waikiki Hotel
La Ronde, 1441 Kapiolani
Maile Room, Kahala Hilton Hotel
The Third Floor, Hawaiian Regent
Top of the Ilikai, 1777 Ala Moana Boulevard
Chez Michel, 2126B Kalakaua
Michel's, Colony Surf

Polynesian

Don the Beachcomber, Waikiki Beachcomber, 2300 Kala-
kaua Avenue
Tahitian Lanai, The Waikikian, 1811 Ala Moana Boulevard
Waioli Tea Room, 3016 Oahu Avenue

Seafood

Fisherman's Wharf, 1009 Ala Moana Boulevard
Nick's Fishmarket, Waikiki Gateway Hotel, 2070 Kalakaua
Avenue
Orson's, Ward Warehouse, 1050 Ala Moana Boulevard

For more ideas on where to dine, read the free *Hawaii Tourist News*, the *Waikiki Beach Press*, or the *Snooper*, then telephone to find out if your choice is accessible.

## MINITOUR 1

WHAT YOU'LL DO

- Tour Paradise Park.
- Lunch at Waioli Tea Room and see Robert Louis Stevenson's grass shack.

HOW YOU'LL DO IT

- Cab from hotel to Paradise Park, 3737 Manoa Road.
- Cab from the Park a half mile to Waioli Tea Room, 3016 Oahu Avenue.
- Cab from the Tea Room to your hotel.

THINGS TO KNOW

- Paradise Park open 9:30 A.M. to 5:30 P.M. Admission $3.50/ $2.
\* - Lunch served at Waioli Tea Room 11:00 A.M. to 2:00 P.M.; tea served from 8:00 A.M. to 4:00 P.M. Reservations advised. Closed Sunday.

RESTROOMS †

- Paradise Park

\* Indicates restriction in time of visit.
$___/$___ indicates adult/child admission fees.
† All sites listed under "Restrooms" offer accessible facilities with wide stall doors and grab bars unless otherwise indicated.

As you might have suspected, a number of roads lead from the bustle of Waikiki to the idyllic Hawaii you've imagined of bamboo forests, lush valleys, mountain waterfalls, bright flowers, and exotic birds. One such road even leads to the proverbial little grass shack. It's Manoa Road in the lush Manoa Valley, once a retreat for Hawaiian royalty and today a garden of lovely homes shaded by flowering trees. In its heart, set around a jungle of hanging vines that was ancient when the first Polynesians discovered the islands, is Paradise Park, a jungle and forest setting bright with the flutter of hundreds of rare birds.

As if the birds, flowers, tropical forests, and ancient jungles weren't enough, the grounds of the Waioli Tea Room, just down the road, shelter an 1880s vintage grass hut supposedly inhabited by Robert Louis Stevenson, who was a guest of the young Princess Kaiulani. And all this is but ten minutes driving time, four and a half miles, from Waikiki!

To get beautifully lost in old Hawaii for a morning or afternoon, begin or end with lunch at the charming **Waioli Tea Room,** built in 1922 by the Salvation Army as part of a training program for their young women in the arts of cooking, baking, and gracious living. One of Hawaii's oldest restaurants, the Tea Room is famed for its good food, including a help-yourself salad bar, Oriental and Hawaiian dishes, and homemade baked goods like mango bread, carrot bread, and macadamia nut brownies. Luncheon is served on the dining lanai where doves fly close in among the border of tree ferns. The grounds are among the island's most gorgeous. There, with assistance, you can see the Stevenson grass shack and the Little Chapel built of native lava rock set among huge leafed monstera and plumeria trees. The gift shop shouldn't be missed. It offers gift packages of poha preserves, chutney, and marinated papaya seed salad dressing. Should you miss lunch, take time for a ramble through the gardens and stop for a glass of Waioli fruit punch in the Coffee Hut.

If you've never been in a jungle before, **Paradise Park** will offer this rare experience and you won't even have to hack your way through! By following the walkway that winds through fifteen acres of gardens overrun with orchids, ginger, jasmine, and hyacinth, you'll come upon a lagoon inhabited by bright pink flamingoes, a waterfall, a pond, and, oh yes, the world's largest free-flight aviary. Inside you'll make nose to beak acquaintance with such feathery friends as rainbow-hued macaws and bright green parrots. Almost every exotic bird that makes the tropical jungles its home will be on hand, some more bold than others as they try to make friends while sitting on your shoulder. Others star in the continuous shows staged in the Kamehameha Amphitheatre. Macaws and cockatoos roller skate, play poker, ride bicycles, and race chariots.

Before leaving you'll want to take a moment to stop by the Photographer's Lanai, where especially friendly tropical birds perch on your shoulder or in your hands for picture taking. If you take someone's photo don't forget to tell them to "watch the little birdie!"

## MINITOUR 2

WHAT YOU'LL DO

* • Visit Foster Botanic Garden.
* • Lunch at and tour the Chinese Cultural Center (closed Sundays).

HOW YOU'LL DO IT

* • Cab from hotel to Foster Garden. Enter at nursery gate on Vineyard Boulevard, halfway between Nuuanu Avenue and River Street.
* • Self-push tour of gardens.
* • Push from nursery gate down Vineyard Boulevard to River Street, then one to two blocks to Cultural Center.
* • Self-push tour of Center.
* • Cab from Center to hotel.

THINGS TO KNOW

* • Foster Garden open 9:00 A.M.–4:00 P.M., no admission charge. There are paved walkways to almost all areas, including the orchid house.
* • Chinese Cultural Plaza open 10:00 A.M.–5:00 P.M., Monday thru Saturday.

RESTROOMS

* • Nonaccessible

* Indicates restriction in time of visit.

Today's a day for incomparable gardens of orchids and 125-year-old trees, for glimpsing the China you thought was thousands of miles away, and for rambling beside a blue river draped in bougainvillea.

Begin with a visit to the **Foster Botanic Garden,** one of the six Honolulu Botanic Gardens located in six different ecological settings. This one is a showcase for tropical flowers and trees, including some varieties of palm that grow nowhere else.

From the nursery entrance on Vineyard Boulevard go beyond the gate and wooden fence to the greenhouse display of hybrid orchids. You'll probably see some shades you never believed existed in nature. Beside the greenhouse, note the baobab tree with trunk so large that in Central Africa it's used for houses, prisons, and water reservoirs. By following the main walkway, you'll reach the entrance, where you can pick up a free self-guided tour folder. Much of the garden is accessible, but not the wild orchid garden nor the Main Terrace where the tallest trees grow. You can, however, see much of the Terrace from the path just below. As you ramble about the gardens look for the cannonball and sausage trees, if you haven't seen them elsewhere. The fruit that dangles from these trees occasioned the strange names.

Also near the entrance you'll want to note the Ceylon Bo tree, propagated from a specimen of the same tree under which Gautama Buddha is said to have sat when he became enlightened. With assistance you'll probably be able to get across the well-trimmed lawn to the garden of poisonous plants and, while you're there, get a look at chocolate, coffee, and cinnamon trees.

You can leave the gardens the same way you entered, then wheel along Vineyard Boulevard to River Street, where you'll see the exotic Kwan Yin Temple. Although you won't be able to get into the temple you can see the elderly Chinese ladies bringing food and flower offerings to tiny outside altars, and sniff the heavy scent of joss.

River Street, heading toward the ocean, follows a blue stream bordered by red-flowering poinciana trees. Along the walkway are canopied benches and tables where Chinese senior citizens play games and talk. If you stop for a moment, one of these friendly old-timers will probably strike up a conversation with you, telling you something about the good old days in this ethnic corner of Honolulu.

In recent times the whole area has changed. An extensive urban renewal project has removed the ramshackle shops and living quarters, replacing them with modern apartments and clean, wide thoroughfares. The $12 million **Chinese Cultural Plaza** is the high-point of the project, a complex of shops and restaurants owned and run by the local Chinese and also the island's Filipino, Japanese, Korean, and South Seas inhabitants.

Before exploring the Center you could roll across the bridge to the old **Toyo Theater.** A side ramp leads up to the theater and provides a good view of a mossy garden of rocks, a pond, and tiny foot bridge. In front of the theater is the Kojima Book Store; you can roll inside and ask for a Japanese comic book or take a look at the karate belt buckles that are for sale.

Just opposite the theater is an entrance into the Center. You'll see the central pavilion where Chinese senior citizens play mahjongg and tin gau as children play their own games on skateboards alongside. Among the shops is the **Chinese Art Center,** with its original brush paintings; the **Dragon Gate Bookshop,** where you can buy lacy paper cuts from China; an exotic health food store; the **Ikebana** florist; and the **Little Pueblo,** featuring American Indian handicrafts.

For lunch you can choose between the **Mongolian Barbeque** restaurant or the **Yang-tze** Restaurant, which specializes in Peking and Shanghai cuisine.

After lunch, call a cab or meet your Handi-Cab beside the Sun Yat Sen statue just outside the restaurant. As you continue back to your hotel, you'll pass through one of Honolulu's oldest areas, seeing such signs as Violet's Lei Stand, Cebu Pool Hall, The Silent Barber Shop—all part of nontourist Hawaii.

## MINITOUR 3

WHAT YOU'LL DO

* • Attend Kodak Hula Show (open Tuesday, Wednesday, and Thursday).

\* Indicates restriction in time of visit.
† All sites listed under "Restrooms" offer accessible facilities with wide stall doors and grab bars unless otherwise indicated.

- Visit Honolulu Zoo.
- Lunch on the terrace of the Kahala Hilton Hotel.

HOW YOU'LL DO IT

- Cab to Kodak Hula Show in Kapiolani Park, next to Band Shell.
- Push from the Show site two blocks to the Honolulu Zoo.
- Cab from the Zoo to the Kahala Hilton Hotel.
- Cab from the Kahala to your hotel.

THINGS TO KNOW

\* • Kodak Hula Show presented free every Tuesday, Wednesday and Thursday morning from 10:00–11:15 A.M. on lawn adjacent to Waikiki Shell. Although other tourists must be on hand thirty to forty-five minutes before the show to get seats, wheelchair visitors are wheeled to front seats just prior to the show's beginning.
- Zoo open 9:00 A.M.–5:00 P.M. No admission charge.
- Hala Terrace of Kahala Hilton open from breakfast thru dinner hours. Dolphins perform daily at 10:30 A.M., 12:30 P.M., and 2:30 P.M.

RESTROOMS †

- Honolulu Zoo
- Kahala Hilton Hotel (restrooms designed for wheelchair users in the planning stage in 1977)

Beautiful island girls in ti-leaf skirts dance, rare Hawaiian nene birds preen under golden shower trees, dolphins leap from a tropical lagoon—exotic sights are on the agenda for this Tuesday, Wednesday, or Thursday morning. It has to be one of these days, since these three weekdays are the only days Kodak puts on their famed free Hula Show in Kapiolani Park. After the show you'll be a shady block or so away from the charming Honolulu Zoo, where you can take a look at the nene, a bird that once was almost extinct but now is doing just fine, thank you. Then after these stops in the park it'll be time for lunch, and since you're only a few miles away from the fabulous Kahala Hilton Hotel and their free dolphin show's on at 2:30, well, who can resist?

Off you go, first to the **Hula Show,** which is held on the lawn next to the Waikiki Shell. Up to 3,000 attend each show, many arriving an hour ahead to get seats. Since there's almost no standing room, one has to have a seat to see the show, which means that if you're traveling with an able friend you'd better be on hand about 9:00 A.M. By being there early you'll have time beforehand to study the Kodak hula book ($2.50), which explains how the hands tell the story. In fact, you can practice. You'll know why the show is so popular when you see the dozens of performers each in an authentic costume representing ancient or modern Hawaii. Young girls in ti-leaf skirts, elderly ladies in mumus, and men and boys dressed as fishermen and warriors tell the story of the islands in song and dance.

After the show, head towards the ocean for about one block to the main entrance of the **Honolulu Zoo.** You may want to take a papaya break at the food stall that you'll pass en route.

As you explore the zoo, reading the signs as you roll past open-air animal habitats, cages, and ponds, you'll begin to sense that you are in a very different kind of zoo. The fact that you have become part of an environment that is as much for the pleasure of the animals as for you will become evident as you reach People Island and see the monkeys watching *you.* What fun! The Zoo pamphlet in your hand now makes more sense as you read about food service and see it broken down into categories for the animals and for man —one lists feeding times, the other tells where the snack bars are. With this new insight you can alternate between watching the children running and tumbling beneath the banyan trees and the young ones in cages swinging on ropes and climbing into tree houses.

As you explore some or all of the two miles of zoo trails, notice the especially fine display of trees and flowers for which the zoo is noted. Show stoppers include the giant banyan tree from India, the golden Kolomona trees, the Monkey Pod or Temple of Shade trees, the Philippine eucalyptus, the blooming star jasmine and spider lilies. If you don't have time for the entire forty-two acres, at least see the monkey island-people island, the new aviary, the rare

Manchurian cranes, the Galapagos tortoise, and the delightful hippo sculpture at the exit.

Continue by cab from the Zoo to the **Kahala Hilton Hotel,** situated between Koko Head and Diamond Head about two miles from Waikiki. Built in a style reminiscent of the grand, airy palaces once inhabited by Hawaiian monarchy, the Kahala Hilton is unique among Hawaii's hotels. The view from the 30-foot-high lobby windows is breathtaking, the surroundings elegant but comfortable.

Follow the oleander-lined driveway to the main entrance, get out at the lobby entrance, and wheel over the handsome parquet teak floors to the reception desk, where you can pick up a copy of the informative walking tour folder. That way you won't miss a thing, not the one-ton crystal chandeliers, the carpets inspired by ancient tapa cloth, or the central copper sculpture.

Continue via elevator to the lagoon level, where you can ramble along one walkway leading to a waterfall tumbling over rocks bordered by heliotrope and sea grapes, and another lined with hawthorn that opens onto a lagoon inhabited by exotic fish and dolphin. If lunch is on your mind, head toward the beachside **Hala Terrace,** from where you can survey this landscape of ocean, waterfall, pond, lagoon, and garden while also watching the comings and goings of man, woman, and dolphins. The dolphins come and go at 12:30 and 2:30 P.M. when they leap into the air for their smelt tidbits—forty pounds of tidbits per day. And you'll have a ringside seat for the show.

## MINITOUR 4

WHAT YOU'LL DO

- Cruise to Pearl Harbor.
- Lunch and shop at the Ward Warehouse.

HOW YOU'LL DO IT

- Handi-Cab from your hotel to Fisherman's Wharf, Kewalo Basin.
- Push from dock across Ala Moana to the Ward Warehouse for self tour.
- Handi-Cab from the Warehouse to your hotel.

THINGS TO KNOW

- Handi-Cab's Pearl Harbor cruise and roundtrip transportation from your hotel offered at a package rate of $9. Reserve twenty-four hours ahead. Depart for the morning cruise at about 10:00 A.M. and return from the Warehouse at about 2:30 P.M.
- Ward Warehouse open 10:00 A.M.–2:00 A.M. daily.

RESTROOMS

- Ward Warehouse (accessible but not especially designed for wheelchair use).

At last, a day to be on the sea, to feel the spray, to study that incredibly blue water at close range, hopefully to see a colorful fish or two—or a school of them.

Several cruise boat companies offer trips to Pearl Harbor, and most are accessible with gangplanks that permit rolling aboard. If assistance is needed, it's plentiful and smiling. One of the best offerings is the package put together by Handi-Cabs that includes a two-hour cruise and roundtrip transportation to and from your hotel for $9. Of course, you'll have to give at least twenty-four hours notice and carefully plan your pickup times. Best plan might be to arrange to be picked up in the morning in time to board the 10:30 A.M. sailing, with a return pickup from the Ward Warehouse at 2:30 or 3:00 P.M. That way you'll have a couple of hours to enjoy the Warehouse complex with its shops and restaurants.

Aboard the comfortable twin-hulled **Pearl Harbor Cruise** company boat, you'll spend two hours at sea and, if you're lucky, will be on a vessel with a glass bottom viewer so you can see the colorful coral beds and exotic fish. As you cruise, your skipper will give you the background on the historic *Arizona* Memorial Monument and point out various ships that you pass that are part of the U.S. Pacific fleet. Best of all, you'll see Honolulu, Waikiki Beach, Diamond Head, the Pali, and much more from your ocean perspective.

When you disembark at the wharf head along the waterfront driveway a few feet in the Diamond Head direction, cross Ala Moana. (There may still be one uncut curb at the street entrance to the

Warehouse where you'll need assistance.) Once inside the **Ward Warehouse** you'll have smooth rolling, as the complex is completely accessible; an elevator will take you to the second level.

Ward Warehouse is unique in that it combines manufacturing and retailing. Zoned for both the making and selling of goods, the Warehouse offers an unusual opportunity to see craftsmen and artists at work making the very things being shown for sale. Depending on the time of year and day you're there, you may see a wood carver making a redwood or teak sign, an artist creating a batik painting, a leatherworker putting the finishing touches on a belt or handbag, a craftsman mitering and nailing moulding together to create a picture frame. The working atmosphere of the Warehouse is reflected in its unusual industrial aesthetic: massive wood trusses, heavy metal braces, wrought iron and rope make up a decor that is both functional and decorative. Notice the sugar mill gears operating on the roof and the abstract design of the children's play area. As you explore, consider your lunch options—perhaps a freshly caught fish at **Orson's,** a down-to-earth cafe overlooking the Kewalo Basin, or a sidewalk sampling of natural food sandwiches, frozen papaya yogurt, or fruit salad.

If you're ready for more adventure, cross Auahi Street to the Ala Moana Farmer's Market, where you can pick up fresh Japanese sushi, Island fruits and fish, or a fragrant ginger lei.

## MINITOUR 5

WHAT YOU'LL DO

- Shop and snack at the Ala Moana Shopping Center.
- Sip and sightsee at twilight from atop La Ronde revolving restaurant.
- Join a poolside barbecue and Hawaiian entertainment party at the Ala Moana Hotel.

HOW YOU'LL DO IT

- Cab from your hotel to the Ala Moana Shopping Center.

† All sites listed under "Restrooms" offer accessible facilities with wide stall doors and grab bars unless otherwise indicated.

- Self-push tour of the center, then to the rooftop La Ronde restaurant in the Ala Moana Building within the Center.
- Wheel with assistance from the center to the Ala Moana Hotel. Use the ramp that links the two, which is accessible from the second level of the parking lot.

THINGS TO KNOW

- Ala Moana Shopping Center open 8:30 A.M.–9:00 P.M. Monday through Friday, 'til 5:30 P.M. on Saturday, 'til 4:00 P.M. on Sundays.
- La Ronde open daily 11:00 A.M.–2:00 P.M., 4:00 P.M.–midnight.
- Poolside barbecues held nightly at the Ala Moana Hotel featuring local talent; $7.95 for buffet with drinks. Make a reservation.

RESTROOMS †

- Ala Moana Shopping Center, lower level behind Hotéi-ya Shop
- Ala Moana Hotel, second floor

There are shopping centers, and then there's the **Ala Moana Shopping Center,** one of the world's largest and most unusual. This center, with its 155 shops, twenty-five-story Ala Moana Building, and its forty-story Ala Moana Hotel, is a city in itself, populated by tens of thousands of islanders and tourists. Bus load after bus load of tourists disembarks at the center throughout the day, some coming back for their second or third visit. There has to be a reason. There are several.

First, the Center is packed with Island families, thus it becomes a living stage on which you can see the real people of the Islands. There's even a playground of sculptures and sand where kids play while their parents shop, and families find the Center an inexpensive way to eat out, as they munch shoyu chicken, poi and moon cakes at outdoor tables under palm trees. On Sunday mornings you can join the locals and tourists for a free show of youngsters between the ages of four and eighteen dancing the Hawaiian hula or fast Tahitian tamure on the Lanai Stage.

Sheer beauty—man-made and natural—also draws people to

the Center. Throughout the three-level complex are trees, flowers, ponds filled with carp, and, in the central mall area, a 160-foot-long stream crossed by arched bridges. The Hawaiian mood is further enhanced with a series of spectacular fountains. One, fifteen feet high, spews forth a thousand gallons of water per minute; another, the Fountain of the Gods, is a column of mosaic tiles in a pool graced by a sculptured flight of gulls.

Art abounds, too, in the galleries that dot the Center, including the **Center Art Gallery,** which recently displayed Salvador Dali's "Lincoln in Dalivision," considered the single most important work in his fifty-year career.

A remarkable variety of modestly priced food also attracts people to the Center, and, oh yes, there are the shops!

Probably nowhere else in the world will you see as many native goods so well displayed. You can literally find anything that's made in Hawaii at the Center, whether it's a frozen luau TV dinner, passion fruit pie, Hawaiian orchid plant, or kukui nut lei. You won't want to miss a look into **Sears Roebuck,** with its unusual Hawaiian specialties, the Japanese department stores, the black coral jewelry at **Tiki Gems,** the Milo wood carvings at **Francis Y,** and the colossal **Foodland Supermarket,** with its exotic specialties from Korea and France and everyplace in between.

If you plan your visit to the Center in the afternoon and have had a late breakfast, you'll probably be inclined to snack your way through paradise. The variety seems to make the snack route the only way to go: consider a sampling of poi and luau pig at the **Poi Hut,** crab in the shell with black bean sauce at **Patti's Chinese Kitchen,** and a slice of passion fruit pie at the **Wonderful World of Pies.** Or for a more restful dining experience, try an Oriental or Hawaiian lunch at **Prince Kuhio's** and see the display of artifacts and Hawaiian monarchs' portraits on display at the restaurant.

By checking your copy of *This Week* or the *Hawaii Tourist News* you'll know if there are any special exhibits or events planned at the Center while you're there. Perhaps you'll catch a Japanese flower arranging exhibit or martial arts demonstration. If your visit is during the summer on a Tuesday or Thursday, try to catch the Hawaiian song and dance performance at 2:00 P.M. on the Lanai Stage.

When you're ready to shift from a close-range view of Hawaii to a broad and open one, head for the Center's **Ala Moana Building.** Take the elevator to the top, then board a second elevator for the final two-floor ascent to **La Ronde.** From your twenty-fifth-floor perch in this oldest revolving restaurant in the United States, you'll see a forever view of mountains, valleys, bay, and surf. The entire revolution takes an hour. If you are there at sunset, you'll see a technicolor view you'll never forget.

As the sun sinks slowly in the west and only ice cubes remain in your glass, you'll probably be ready to continue your tour by wheeling over to the Ala Moana Hotel right next door. Best way to reach the hotel is by descending to the third-floor mall level and taking the ramp that leads from the second floor of the parking lot to the Ala Moana Hotel. Since the ramp to the hotel is a steep one, you'll need assistance.

The **Ala Moana Hotel's** combination nightly barbecue and Hawaiian talent show is surprisingly folksy, not like the usual hotel dinner show. This one really goes native, with islanders themselves joining the party and entertainers ready to have a good time. On a typical evening the songs and dances go on long into the night, long after you've heard almost every Hawaiian song ever written, have sung along, told the story of the hula with your hands, and your cab driver has deposited you at your own "little grass shack" hotel in Waikiki.

## MINITOUR 6

WHAT YOU'LL DO

* • See the exhibits and enjoy the courtyards at the Honolulu Academy of Arts, with lunch at the Garden Cafe.
* • Visit and tour the State Capitol (weekdays only).
  • Tour by cab the grounds of Iolani Palace, the Judiciary Building, King Kamehameha statue, the Kawaiahao Church, and Mission Houses.

* Indicates restriction in time of visit.

† All sites listed under "Restrooms" offer accessible facilities with wide stall doors and grab bars unless otherwise indicated.

HOW YOU'LL DO IT

- Cab from your hotel to the Honolulu Academy of Art, 900 South Beretania Street. Use side entrance on Piikoi Street.
- Cab from the Academy to the State Capitol, Beretania Street ramped entrance.
- Cab from Capitol to hotel via Iolani Palace, Judiciary Building, Kawaiahao Church, Mission Houses.

THINGS TO KNOW

\* • Honolulu Academy of Arts open 10:00 A.M.–4:30 P.M. Tuesday–Saturday, 2:00 P.M.–5:00 P.M. Sunday. Cafe Lanai closed during the summer. Call first to have side door opened or send someone at main entrance to tell receptionist. Lunch reservations a must.
\* • Tours of the State Capitol given weekdays from about 10:00 A.M.–3:00 P.M. Beautiful color booklet available free of charge.

RESTROOMS †

- State Capitol

Tearing yourself away from the beauties of nature to see an art gallery and a federal building may not at first seem like the world's greatest idea. But wait! Even if the gallery weren't renowned and the building stunningly innovative, there'd still be good cause to don your straw hat and roll on. That's because these two buildings are total environments that create a mood and give a sense of old and new Hawaii that can't be found elsewhere.

The **Honolulu Academy of Arts,** built in 1922, was the first building to express a truly Hawaiian style of architecture. The peaked roof, borrowed from the old Polynesian design, and the informal lanais taken from the early missionary houses were combined with Oriental styles to form a unique architectural form.

In contrast, the supremely modernistic **Capitol** is inspired by nature, literally telling the story of the birth of Hawaii in concrete and steel. The building, with its volcanic cone-shaped roof, is set in a reflecting pool symbolizing the formation of the islands from the sea. Columns represent palm trees and a great central court open to the sun and rain has as its focal point a mosaic floor reflecting the changing colors and patterns of shore waters.

To see and fully sense both of these gems and their surrounding neighbors, set aside a morning or afternoon, beginning or ending with lunch at the Academy's **Cafe Lanai.** In this charming restaurant you'll choose from a menu of lovingly prepared specialties such as peanut salad with poppy seed dressing, carrot soup, and sesame cheese biscuits.

While at the Academy you'll want to see some of the thirty exhibition galleries displaying a renowned collection of Oriental and Western art. Of particular note are the Chinese ceramics from the neolithic period, the relief carvings from India, Buddhist and Shinto art of medieval Japan, Chinese furniture of the Ming and Ch'ing dynasties, and European master oils including one by Monet.

Between your appreciation of these art objects, take time to enjoy the Chinese Court, patterned after a Peking garden, the lovely Spanish Court, and the sitting rooms with their fine old furnishings and dramatic fresh flower arrangements.

At the Capitol you'll see more artwork in the governor's and lieutenant governor's offices, which are on the conducted tour. You'll also have a glimpse of the Moon chandelier in the Senate, made of polished aluminum and nautilus shells. But best of all is the great courtyard itself, open to the sky. The mosaic by famed Japanese artist Tadashi Sato is called "Aquarius." Notice, too, the charming Marisol statue of Father Damien, which faces the mountain at the entrance. While you're at the Capitol, be sure to pick up the beautiful color booklet that's free of charge.

As you ramble around the Capitol courtyard, you'll see Hawaii's most historic buildings in the ocean direction. When you're ready to leave, ask your cab driver to drive around the Iolani Palace, where once kings and queens and nobles strolled along walkways and balconies. Then continue along King Street for a look at the bronze statue of King Kamehameha the Great, the Judiciary Building (originally designed to be a palace), the Kawaiahao Church where many of Hawaii's nobility are buried, and the adjoining Mission Houses, three restored missionary homes. (None of these buildings is accessible.)

Although you'd need assistance, you could push from the Capitol to the Iolani Bandstand behind the Iolani Palace on Richards Street. That prospect may be tempting indeed if you hear the lively Royal Hawaiian Band playing, which it does each Friday at noon.

## TOUR 1

WHAT YOU'LL DO

- Overlook the green sea in the horseshoe-shaped crater of Hanauma Bay.
- Stop to see spouting Halona Blowhole.
* • Visit Sea Life Park (closed Mondays).
* • Lunch at Haiku Gardens (closed Mondays) or Polynesian Cultural Center (closed Sundays).
* • Visit to Polynesian Cultural Center (closed Sundays).
- Visit to Kahuku Sugar Mill.
- Stop at Dole Pineapple Pavilion to buy a pineapple.
* • Dine at the Willows Restaurant (closed Sundays).

HOW YOU'LL DO IT

- Drive along the windward side of the island from Waikiki to Haleiwa, then return to Honolulu via the inner island highway.
- Optional detour from coast highway along Haiku Road to Haiku Gardens.
- Drive from Waikiki via Ala Wai Boulevard, crossing the McCully Street Bridge. Turn right on Kapiolani, following it five blocks to Hausten Street and the Willows Restaurant, 901 Hausten Street.

THINGS TO KNOW

- Handicapped parking a few feet from the lookout over Hanauma Bay.
- Good view of Blowhole from Halona Lookout.

* Indicates restriction in time of visit.
$___/$___ indicates adult/child admission fees.
† All sites listed under "Restrooms" offer accessible facilities with wide stall doors and grab bars unless otherwise indicated.

*  • Sea Life Park open daily 10:00 A.M.–5:00 P.M., except Monday. Admission $3/$1.50.
*  • Polynesian Cultural Center in Laie on North Shores open daily 10:00 A.M.–7:00 P.M. except Sundays. Admission $4.25/$2.25. For a schedule of events and show or dinner reservations, call 923–1861.
   • Kahuku Sugar Mill open 10:00 A.M.–6:00 P.M. Two-and-one-half-hour tour shows sugar-making process, but only first half of tour is accessible. Cost $3.50/$2.25.
*  • Haiku Gardens open daily except Monday.
*  • Willows Restaurant open daily except Sunday. Lunch from 11:30 A.M., dinner from 5:30 P.M.

RESTROOMS †

• Sea Life Park
• Laie-Maloo Beach, across from Polynesian Cultural Center
• Polynesian Cultural Center (restrooms accessible but not designed for wheelchair use).

The scenery changes as you drive from Waikiki Beach over Diamond Head to Makapuu Point and the forty-four miles of roadway that curls around the windward side of Oahu to Haleiwa. On this most delightful of drives you'll pass from volcanic formations of stark beauty and geysers of sea water to a curving coastline bordering the sea. On the lands fronting the coral beaches with pounding surf or quiet bays you'll see picturesque towns, grazing cattle, lush fields of sugar cane, and forests of breadfruit, papaya, and coconut palm. Fruit stands sell bananas and pineapples along this route. Vibrant hibiscus blooms and flowering poinciana and plumeria trees contrast against green mountains and blue sky. As you turn off the coastline drive at Haleiwa, you'll bisect the island, passing en route endless fields of pineapple.

The drive can be made in several hours, but the trip could take days or weeks, depending on the number of stops and how long you stop. With a good eight-hour day, however, you should have plenty of time to enjoy a look at Hanauma Bay and the spectacle of Blowhole, with longer stops at Sea Life Park, the Polynesian Cultural Center, and the Kahuku Sugar Mill.

Begin by driving along Diamond Head Road and Kahala Avenue to the lookout at Diamond Head. Then, following H-1 to the Kalanianaole Highway, continue past Koko Head to **Hanauma Bay,** a horseshoe-shaped crater of pale green water bordered by white sand and palm trees. You can roll to an observation area overlooking the bay or drive down to the water's edge for a closer look.

From the Bay you'll continue to the **Halona Blowhole** and then around Makapuu Point to Sea Life Park.

**Sea Life Park,** beautifully situated at the base of 1000-foot lava cliffs overlooking Makapuu Beach, is Hawaii's greatest paid attraction, drawing over half a million visitors yearly. You'll find out why as you tour the sixty-two-acre site, with its displays of Hawaiian marine life in completely natural settings. Highlight for most is seeing a living coral reef three fathoms beneath the surface of the water. Via a circular ramp you view a 300,000-gallon glass tank inhabited by hundreds of marine creatures, each living at depths it prefers. Reef sharks glide, eels undulate, crustacea scurry, turtles plod—the watery scene filled with thousands of marine creatures is almost frantic. To make matters even more hectic, a scuba diver slips over the side several times a day to hand feed the sea creatures.

Also to be seen are performing porpoise and whales, penguins, seals and sea lions, a lagoon of giant turtles, and a feeding pool filled with friendly sea lions and seals looking for a handout.

Along the thirty-five-mile stretch between Sea Life Park and the Polynesian Cultural Center, you'll pass a dozen beach parks, points, landings, and lookouts. You could quite easily stop at every other turn and see the ocean from a different viewpoint, sometimes with an island in the shape of a chinaman's hat (which it's called) and sometimes without.

You can lunch at the Polynesian Cultural Center or in Kaneohe at the **Haiku Gardens,** where you'll eat in a restaurant overlooking a vast garden of eucalyptus and banana trees, lily ponds, and bamboo groves.

The next best thing to a cruise through the South Seas is a stop at Laie and the **Polynesian Cultural Center.** Here in a garden setting of lagoons and waterways you travel to seven Polynesian islands—villages of grass huts, bamboo houses, tribal halls, and picket fence–enclosed fortresses. The villages, constructed in native fashion, represent the people of Fiji, Hawaii, Samoa, Tonga, Tahiti, the Marquesas, and the Maoris of New Zealand. You can look inside the village buildings, around which young native people of each island demonstrate their crafts as they make tapa cloth, pound taro root, weave baskets of lauhala, carve canoes, and fashion wooden kava bowls.

The Center, built by the Mormon Church, provides work for Pacific islander students attending the Brigham Young–Hawaii University. Over 150 of these Polynesian students work their way through college by singing, dancing, and sharing their cultures with visitors at the Center. A show of authentic songs and dances is presented twice each evening in the 1000-seat amphitheater and a Long Canoe Pageant each day at 3:30 P.M.

The **Kahuku Sugar Mill,** beyond the Center, was built in 1890 to process sugar cane, closed in 1971, and reopened as a visitor attraction in 1976. Recipient of the 1977 National Trust President's Award, the Mill is a noteworthy historic preservation. Only the first half of the tour is accessible, but even if you don't take the tour you can, for no charge, explore the grounds, which are accessible. From the base of the mill you can look up to see the huge flywheels and gears, crusher rolls, centrifuges, the cane washing apparatus, and an 1870 vintage steam locomotive juice wagon. There's also a network of accessible shops housed in the old buildings. If you're a coffee lover, try a cup of Kona coffee, which is sold at one of the stands.

From the Mill, your route continues to Haleiwa, where you turn onto Highway 82 for the twenty-five-mile trip back to Honolulu. Along this route you pass through miles of pineapple fields. About a third of the way back you will come to the **Dole Pineapple Pavilion,** a veritable pineapple supermarket. Fresh field pineapples, pineapples cut into chunks, and pineapple juice are dispensed with the efficiency of a Manhattan superette. But the fragrance is nice, and so is the fact that you can roll out the back door to pick your own pineapple right from the field.

With pineapples in hand, you'll probably reach your Waikiki Beach hotel in plenty of time for sunset libations. Then, since you have a car, you might plan on dinner at one of Hawaii's most romantic restaurants, the **Willows.** Open dining lanais overlook carp-filled ponds and tropical gardens fringed by dreamy willow trees. You can sample Hawaii's popular mahimahi fish or choose from a good menu of shrimp curry, seafood salads, and entrees—topped off with the restaurant's famed coconut cream pie.

By making this windward drive and seeing the sights suggested in the minitours, you've seen the best of Hawaii—with one exception. You've missed the drive along Nuuanu Valley through forests of bamboo, ginger, and fern to the 1207-foot **Pali Lookout,** with its magnificent view of the Kailua–Kaneohe Bay area. Only a romantic would consider it, but you could dash up to the Pali Lookout in the morning before turning the car in—it opens very early! If not in the early morning, go when the Pali calls, whether it's by cab or Handi-Cab or when you come to Hawaii again. You must have a reason to come back and what better one?

### Beach Park Restrooms

(All are wheelchair-accessible, with wide doors and grab bars.)

Ala Moana Beach Park
Haleiwa-Alii Beach Park
Hauula Beach Park
Hanauma Bay Beach Park
Kaaawa Beach Park
Kahana Bay Beach Park
Kahe Point Beach Park
Kailua Beach Park
Kainoa Beach Park
Kapiolani Park Beach Center
Keehi Lagoon Beach Park
Koko Head District Park
Kuliouou Beach Park
Maili Beach Park
Mokuleia Beach Park
Nanakuli Beach Park
Nuuanu Valley Park
Pokai Bay Beach Park

Pupukea Beach Park
Sandy Beach Park
Swanzy Beach Park
Waialae Beach Park
Waialua Beach Park
Waimanalo Beach Park
Waimea Bay Beach Park

## Other Accessible Attractions

Amfax Towers (lobby art exhibit)
Hawaiian Village Dome (for evening entertainment)
Honolulu Aquarium
Kahala Shopping Mall
King's Alley & Heritage Theatre
Mekkiki Christian Church (a Japanese samurai palace)
Pine Grove Village, on Kalanianaoli Highway
St. Augustine Chapel

INTRODUCING
*Rollin' On* adviser, wheeler Lowell Grant

*Title:* Member of Mayor's Committee on Handicapped, Chairman
of Barrier Free Design and Transportation
*Telephone number:* (808) 533–2794
*Hometown:* Honolulu
*Favorite tourist site:* Paradise Park
*Hidden corner:* Nuuanu Valley
*Rendezvous:* La Ronde or the Halekulani Lani
*Offbeat restaurant:* Blue Hawaii
*Place for music:* lobby of the Hawaiian Regent Hotel at the cock-
tail hour
*View:* from Round Top Drive, Mt. Tantalus
*Natural wonder:* Diamond Head
*Museum:* Honolulu Academy of Arts
*Ramble:* along River Street bordering the Chinese Cultural Center
*Non-tourist destination:* Ala Moana Farmers Market
*Offbeat experience:* a free ride by Navy boat to Pearl Harbor

*Traditional restaurant:*  The Willows or the Waioli Tea Room
*Low-cost restaurant:*  Penny's at the Ala Moana Shopping Center
     or the Flamingo Chuck Wagon on Kapiolani Boulevard
*Ice cream shop:*  Farrells at the Ala Moana Shopping Center
*Reading suggestion:  Hawaii* by James Mitchner
*Place to get a wheelchair repaired:*  Grant Wheelchair Repair Co.
*Tip on having a great time in Honolulu:* Buy a palm frond hat and
     relax beside the water where you can also people-watch. Go
     to a luau put on by a local church group. Buy a flower lei and
     give it to a friend. Try some poi, smell some Wicked Wahini
     perfume, sip a tall, cool drink with a pineapple swizzle stick.

# 7

# New York

You simply must see New York at least once!

You must, even though you know New York has its problems and that you may share a few. You want to sense this city at last: its variety and disparity, its outrageous glamour and its seedy despair, its constantly renewed determination to be the most powerful, the most exciting, the most total megalopolis in the world. For if you were to list every adjective known to man, those words would describe New York.

New York is everything. It is a smorgasbord where sights, pleasures, and experiences are set out for your savoring. All you must do is choose—or stay forever to see and do it all:

- to rendezvous with the Statue of Liberty to see, as if from her mild eyes, the "sea washed sunset gates . . . beside the golden door."
- to know first-hand the hectic beat of our nation's financial heart, which you discover on your own amidst a crazy quilt of narrow streets in a jumble of granite and chrome.
- to find the New York of yesterday that goes on living today within the sensual muraled walls and rooftop gardens of that city within a city, Rockefeller Center.
- to share the sunlit waters of the East River from the United Nation's rose garden with a Buddhist delegate in a saffron robe.
- to ramble up Fifth Avenue past the glitter of Tiffany's and

the joys of F.A.O. Schwarz to the splashing fountain and hansom cabs at the entrance to Central Park.

- to forget time in the cool marble halls of the Metropolitan Museum of Art, lost in the ancient civilization of Egypt or in the intrigue of an eighteenth-century French court.
- to conquer Manhattan once and for all with a I-have-it-in-the-palm-of-my-hand cruise around the little twelve-by-three-mile island as sunset washes the jagged skyline in a glow of pink.

Finding the best of New York takes careful planning or the opposite—an open, eager heart ready to find the New York that is gracious and kind. Views by wheelers of New York vary: one says, "It's the friendliest place in the world, a place where I've always gotten a cab within five minutes and felt strangers were eager to be of help." Another native New York wheelchair user says simply, "It's a challenge—always."

To be ready for the best—but also prepared for anything—it can't hurt to avoid questionable areas, to be where other people are as a form of protection by numbers, to call ahead for cabs to be picked up at the place you're leaving, and to show your appreciation for extra service by generous tips.

Whatever you do, don't miss a visit to New York's first building designed to be totally accessible. It's the stunning Citicorp Center at Lexington Avenue and 49th Street, a city-block-square complex that includes a skyscraper office building, a glass-roofed atrium shopping and dining mall, and one of the most beautiful churches to be erected in Manhattan in this century. You'll roll into the center from Lexington Avenue, passing St. Peter's Lutheran Church with its chapel designed by sculptress Louise Nevelson. Inside the three-level atrium you'll have access to thirty shops and restaurants representing the many ethnic origins of the people of New York. Among the international restaurants are Alfredo's of Rome, Auberge Suisse, Avgerinos for Greek cuisine, Hungaria and Les Tournebroches.

## Planning Your Trip

Get together all the information you can about Manhattan, and while you're at it, round up an able friend to accompany you. This may be the only city where you'll need assistance every time you roll out of your hotel. Curb cuts are almost nonexistent, and you can't count on driveways in most areas. If you're a jock, you'll be able to jump the curbs that most often are low, but otherwise you'll find yourself asking for assistance at every corner.

Two publications give you details about accessible sites, restaurants, and other facilities in New York. One is *The New York City Guide,* put out by the Easter Seal Society. To obtain it send your request to the Society at 2 Park Avenue, Suite 1815, New York, N.Y. 10016. The Institute of Rehabilitation Medicine publishes *Access New York,* which you can obtain by writing to the Institute at New York University Medical Center, 400 East 34th Street, New York, N.Y. 10016. Include 50¢. This publication lists accessible restaurants by street so that you can make your selections near your hotel or in the area of the attractions you'll be seeing.

To supplement this list, native New York wheelers point to these accessible restaurants as being unique New York experiences:

Algonquin Hotel's Rose Room and Oak Room 59 West 46th Street
Charlie Brown's, Pan Am Building
P. J. Clarke's, 915 Third Avenue
The Cookery, 21 University Place (at 8th Street)
Four Seasons, 99 East 52nd Street
La Crepe, 57 West 56th Street
Luchow's, 114 East 14th Street (2 steps)
Mama Leone's, 239 West 48th Street (ask for special door)
Pete's Tavern, 66 Irving Place
Promenade Cafe, Rockefeller Center
Rainbow Room, Rockefeller Center
Rossoff's, 147 West 43rd Street
Rumpelmayer's, 50 Central Park South
Russian Tea Room, 150 West 57th Street
Tavern on the Green, Central Park
Top of the Sixes, 666 Fifth Avenue
Trattoria, 200 Park Avenue

Write ahead for maps and literature, dispensed free of charge by the New York Convention and Visitors Bureau, 90 East 42nd

Street, New York, N.Y. 10017. Also you may want to write for the accessibility guide put out by Lincoln Center's Public Information Department, 1865 Broadway, New York, N.Y. 10023.

Of course you'll want to attend a play, opera, concert, or dance performance while in this theatrical enclave. A good way to go about getting tickets is to buy the *New York Times* to find out what's playing, the name of the theater, its address, and the prices being charged. Write requesting your tickets, specify that you're in a wheelchair, and include a check and a self-addressed and stamped envelope.

Except for theaters at Lincoln Center most are minimally accessible, but some offer special access. The only way to find out in advance is by writing and asking at the time you request tickets.

What's the best time of year for a visit to New York? Summer can be very hot, but it also can be delightful, and during the summer Central Park becomes the stage for concerts and plays, including Shakespeare. More entertainment is offered at the South Street Seaport. Fall is the New York theater season, with Lincoln Center in full swing and a flurry of shows all over town. In the spring Rockefeller Center's Channel Gardens blossom with new floral displays every few weeks, including a dazzle of Easter lilies for that holiday. During that season artists set up shop around Washington Square for their annual outdoor art exhibit.

What to bring along on your trip to New York? Plenty of money, of course. Also your nicest clothes, as few cities are more chic. Even salesgirls and clerks have that up-to-the-minute fashion magazine look. But don't bring too many clothes, leave space in your suitcase for that special New York City purchase, that something of quality and high fashion that will tell everyone you meet where you've been.

**How to Get There**

New York is served by three airports, a bus terminal, and two railroad stations.

Airports are Kennedy International, LaGuardia, and Newark International. All are accessible, with special wheelchair-accessible restrooms. Taxi fare from Kennedy to mid-town, 20 miles, is about

$18.50, including bridge tolls. From La Guardia it's about $8, and the same from Newark if you join other passengers in the cab—otherwise it's around $20.

The Port Authority Bus Terminal at Eighth Avenue and 40th Street is the terminus for Greyhound, Trailways, and a host of other more regional carriers. The Terminal is accessible and offers restrooms that are accessible to wheelchair users.

Amtrak trains from Chicago, Washington, Boston, plus points north, south, and west arrive at either Grand Central or Penn Station, both a short cab ride from mid-Manhattan hotels. Accessible restrooms are available at both stations. At Penn Station wheelchair users can enter on 31st Street and use the loading zone elevator.

## Getting Around

As mentioned previously, New York is low on curb cuts and there aren't many driveways either. So to get around you have to jump curbs, ask for assistance, or have a friend pushing. The itineraries outlined here are based on the supposition you'll have assistance, which accounts for the use of *wheel* as opposed to *push* under the "How You'll Do It" section.

Cabs are plentiful—there are over 12,000 in New York City—but relatively expensive at a basic 75¢ the minute you get in plus 70¢ per mile. But, considering you will be making only a few trips over two miles, the total cost may be less than other cities. Among the several cab companies that are accustomed to carrying wheelchair passengers is the surprisingly affable Queens 2-Way Cab Company (576–0707). If you'll specify you're in a chair, they'll put that information into their coded dispatch so that drivers who are trained to assist you can pick up the call.

You may be surprised at how helpful New Yorkers and the visitors to New York are when you do need assistance. And with a nice tip to your hotel doorman each time he gives you a hand, you should be assured of efficient cab transfers.

A consideration that may influence your getting around is the dearth of wheelchair-accessible restrooms in New York City. Unfortunately you can't count on any restaurant having appropriate facilities, and the tourist attractions that do are few in number. The itineraries here have been planned around restroom stops, except for evening activities, which offer few possibilities. This is one of the problems mentioned in connection with visiting New York. The only answer is to know where you can find standard wheelchair facilities. Here is the most up-to-date list that could be obtained of those facilities, with or without grab bars, that have stall doors opening to 32 inches or wider:

Asia House Gallery, 112 East 64th Street

Battery Park, southern tip Manhattan

East Side Airlines Terminal, First Avenue and 30th Street

Grand Central Station, 42nd Street between Lexington and Park avenues

Jewish Museum, 92nd Street at Fifth Avenue (ramp plus 3 steps)

Lincoln Center, Broadway and 64th Street

Merrill Lynch, 165 Broadway

Metropolitan Museum of Art, Fifth Avenue and 82nd Street

Museum of Natural History, Central Park West at 79th Street. Use ramp under main staircase.

Museum of the City of New York, Fifth Avenue and 105th Street. Use 104th Street entrance.

New York Stock Exchange, 20 Broadway

Port Authority Bus Terminal, Eighth Avenue and 40th Street

St. Bartholomew's Church, Park Avenue between 50th and 51st streets

Statue of Liberty, Liberty Island

Temple Emanu-el, Fifth Avenue and 65th Street. Use entrance at 1 East 65th Street.

Saks Fifth Avenue, Fifth Avenue at 57th Street

World Trade Center, 1 Liberty Place

## Where to Stay

Here comes problem number two, or is it number three or four? With 100,000 first class hotel rooms, one might think there would be some designed for wheelchair users. Not so. Maybe because most hotels are older. However, there are some that are accessible and that also have guest rooms with wide doors into the room and into the bathroom. Among these hotels (with bathroom door dimensions indicated) are:

> Berkshire, 21 East 52nd Street, 29 inches
> Biltmore, Madison Avenue at 43rd Street, 27 inches
> Gramercy Park, Lexington at 21st Street, 27 inches
> New York Hilton, 1335 Avenue of Americas and 54th Street, 32 inches
> Roger Smith, 501 Lexington Avenue and 47th Street, 28½ inches

Other possibilities include:

> Holiday Inn, 440 West 57th Street
> Howard Johnson Motor Lodge, Eighth Avenue and 50th Street
> Marriott Essex House, 160 Central Park South
> Statler Hilton, 401 Seventh Avenue

Of all these the modern **New York Hilton** is superbly situated within a few blocks of many of the top attractions and has Rockefeller Center as its neighbor. The 2153-room hotel offers a steak house, continental restaurant, coffeeshop, and a busy lobby ideal for people-watching. Less expensive but also in a convenient sightseeing area is the 1917 vintage **Roger Smith Hotel,** which has been refurbished. Rooms are large and nicely furnished. If the 28″ wide main elevator is a little snug for your chair, the freight elevator just a few feet away offers a 32″ entrance.

The **Doral Inn** at 49th Street and Lexington Avenue is the former Belmont Plaza, which underwent a multimillion dollar modernization. This beautiful, mid-priced hotel is completely accessible with sliding doors, wide elevators and level access to restaurants. The only problem is that the bathroom doors are only 22″ wide after the door is removed; the management will remove the bathroom door upon request.

### What You'll See and Do

Here is a selection of the major sights and experiences—a smorgasbord of New York. You could as well cover half of what each

daily itinerary suggests, with the remainder of the day left for shopping, eating, and the planning of evening tours to famous night
spots. You could spend a half day in Greenwich Village, but be
careful, as it's gone downhill in recent years. You could trek to the
Empire State Building, but the observation tower is not accessible.
You could join the scurry at Herald Square and shop in the biggest
department store anywhere, Macy's. There's so much more, and to
help you decide we have included a supplemental list of accessible
sightseeing options. Be sure to read the *New York Times*, *New
York* magazine, and *Cue* for timely ideas. And if you have a special question or problem, call your friends at the Easter Seal Society—(212) 532–8830—asking for Eileen Healey, who is the
official New York adviser to *Rollin' On*.

## TOUR 1

### WHAT YOU'LL DO

- Cruise to the Statue of Liberty.
- Visit the New York Stock Exchange.
- Tour Federal Hall.
- Visit Trinity Church.
- Lunch at World Trade Center with ascent to 107th-floor ob-
  servation deck.
- Visit to South Street Seaport Museum and tour of New Fulton
  Market.
- Dinner in or near hotel.

### HOW YOU'LL DO IT

- Cab from hotel to Battery Park, State and Water streets.
- Push five short blocks from Battery Park to the New York
  Stock Exchange.
- Push across street to the Federal Hall, Pine Stret entrance.
- Push two blocks to Trinity Church, 74 Trinity Place.
- Push three block to World Trade Center, 1 Liberty Street.
- Cab from World Trade Center to South Street Seaport, Pier
  16.

$___/$___ indicates adult/child admission fees.
† All sites listed under "Restrooms" offer accessible facilities with wide
stall doors and grab bars unless otherwise indicated.

- Push across street to New Fulton Market, South and Fulton streets.
- Push one block to attractions on Front and Water streets.
- Cab from South Street area to your hotel.

THINGS TO KNOW

- Statue of Liberty boats leave on the hour from 9:00 A.M.–4:00 P.M. Fare is $1.50/50¢. The trip takes twenty minutes each way.
- New York Stock Exchange theater, museum exhibit open 10:00 A.M.–4:00 P.M. daily. Free.
- Federal Hall open 9:00 A.M.–4:30 P.M. Free.
- World Trade Center 107th-floor observation deck open 9:30 A.M.–9:30 P.M. daily.
- South Street Seaport open 12:00 noon–6:00 P.M. daily. Donations.
- New Fulton Market open 11:00 A.M.–6:00 P.M. weekdays, 11:00 A.M.–7:00 P.M. weekends.
- South Street Seaport Museum open daily 12:00 noon–6:00 P.M.

RESTROOMS †

- Battery Park
- Statue of Liberty
- New York Stock Exchange
- World Trade Center

Begin your first day in New York with a pilgrimage to America's most symbolic structure, the **Statue of Liberty,** reached by ferry from **Battery Park.** Ask the cab driver to let you out at the entrance closest to the ferry boat ticket office. You can, if time and energy permit, explore the Park, with its Marine Memorial and the round brownstone Castle Clinton, built in 1811 as a defense against the British; later it became for a time the nation's principal immigrant depot.

The twenty-minute ferry ride to Liberty Island will invite contemplation of the meaning of the Statue and also encourage appreciation of the herculean task the sculptor had in assembling the 151-foot masterpiece.

You can disembark on Liberty Island and tour the new American Museum of Immigration and read the familiar words of the poetic tribute written by Emma Lazarus: "Give me your tired, your poor, your huddled masses yearning to breathe free." Take a look at the Statue of Liberty Gift Shop, an authorized U.S. National Park Service concession with distinctive gifts and souvenirs.

If you get off on Liberty Island, you'll find yourself back at Battery Park an hour and forty minutes later; if you stay aboard the ferry for the return trip, you'll be back in forty minutes.

From Battery Park you can wheel two short blocks up Pearl Street to Broad Street to see a rare example of a complete block of early buildings that have been restored. Notice Fraunces Tavern, an eighteenth-century colonial brick residence reconstructed in 1907 that now serves as a restaurant and museum (inaccessible).

Continue three short blocks along Broad Street to the ornate **New York Stock Exchange,** which together with Federal Hall across the street best represents the astounding growth of this financial heart of America. From this vantage you can see along Wall Street the major institutions that have created much of the wealth and power of our nation. You are at the center of America's—and the world's—financial empires.

Go to the second-floor museum, where you'll see a film on the Exchange, tour displays by some of America's major companies, and have your questions answered by guides. Notice the historic display, which includes an 1867 New York Stock Exchange ticker, and take a moment to look at the gift counter, which sells bull and bear ties. Unfortunately the gallery overlooking the Exchange is inaccessible, due to steep stairs and a narrow door.

From the Exchange roll across the street to **Federal Hall,** noting the impressive statue of George Washington on the front steps. Enter around the back on Pine Street where there's a ramp. In this accessible building you'll see a superb audiovisual exhibit on the city's early history. You'll also find out about this historic building, a national memorial that was recently reopened after renovation. The building was constructed in 1842 as the U.S. Customs House on the site of the original Federal Hall, where George Washington took his oath of office and where Congress passed the Bill of Rights in 1789.

Continue along Wall Street two short blocks to **Trinity Church,** the spiritual home of the old Anglican aristocracy. It was chartered in 1697 by King William III. The present structure is the third to stand on this site. The overpowering monument to martyrs of the American Revolution that you see on the northeast corner was erected to prevent the city from running Pine Street through the cemetery; a statute prevents the removal of any public monument for the purpose of highway improvement.

Passing through the churchyard, where you can look for the tombstones of Alexander Hamilton and Robert Fulton, continue along Trinity Street to the right, noting the fantasy of Gothic detail on the U.S. Realty Building at 111 Trinity Street. When you reach Liberty Street, stop for a rest in Marine Midland Plaza, noting the Noguchi sculpture, a large red cube.

You're across the street from the **World Trade Center.** As you tilt your head further and further back trying to see the tops of the two 110-story towers, keep an eye out for the fabulous window washing machine that automatically washes five stories of windows in one minute—there are 21,800 windows in each tower.

Wheel on over and begin your exploration of this six-acre city of 50,000 workers and 80,000 daily visitors.

Entering the Liberty Street lobby you can ramble over the lush blue carpets past walls of glass and shiny mylar to elevators that will whisk you to the enclosed observation gallery on the 107th floor. From this vantage you overlook New York Harbor, Manhattan, the New Jersey Turnpike, the Brooklyn Bridge, and the Atlantic Ocean. Pointing out the major sites are captions beneath many of the 232 windows. (The 110th-floor outdoor observation area can be reached only by escalator.)

Down to earth on the concourse level you can explore the numerous shops, including F. A. O. Schwarz, New York's most famous toy emporium. You can also see an exhibition at the U.S. Customs House.

For lunch choose between such concourse-level eateries as the **Market Bar** or **Big Kitchen** or ascend to the **Forty-fourth-floor cafeteria,** with its narrow windows overlooking the city and harbor. This unusual luncheon spot features a blue-sky ceiling with white clouds that matches the T-shirts that the cafeteria personnel wear. As for food, it's reasonable and imaginative, particularly the goodies listed under the "chocolate-break" menu.

From the World Trade Center, take a cab a dozen blocks to the **South Street Seaport Museum,** getting out at Pier 16. This indoor, outdoor museum is being restored to bring to life again those mid-nineteenth-century days when this was one of the world's great sailing ship ports. During the 1850s, the high noon of New York's maritime empire, this waterfront was crowded with coasters or larger class vessels bound for Africa, India, China, South America, the Orient, and Europe. Barrels, sacks, boxes, hampers, bales, and hogsheads crammed the quays and burst forth from every ware-house. Sail makers, riggers, figurehead carvers, merchants, sailors, captains, and draymen filled the busy streets and wharves.

Today old brick is being steamed clean, elegant Victorian shop fronts are being renovated according to old drawings—the area again is becoming a market of goods, ideas, and people. You can see the exteriors of such historic ships as the *Peking*, *Ambrose*, and *Howard* moored at Pier 16 and enjoy the watery scene from be-neath the awnings of an open-air snack bar.

Although the streets are quite rough in spots, determined wheel-ers can roll from Pier 16 across the street to the **New Fulton Market,** with its shops and nineteenth-century bar, which now dispenses clams, oysters, and fried fish. Note the huge globe beside the bar, a safe salvaged from an old ship. Among the shops to explore are those specializing in needlecraft, nautical antiques, African fabric and jewelry, and gourmet coffee and spices. You may also catch artisans at work: glass blowers and potters.

Across the street at the **Visitors' Center** you can see a film ori-enting you to the area and view a tugboat exhibit. Notable in the museum is a carved and painted figurehead, probably of a French naval officer.

A number of other interesting sites are within a block of the Museum and may be accessible by the time you make your visit. These include Bowne & Company Stationers and Printing Museum, the Sail Ship Model Gallery, Steamship Model Gallery, Museum Art Gallery, the Book and Chart Store, which is heralded by a sextant above the door, and a small park marked by a monument to those lost at sea aboard the *Titanic.*

While you're rolling around, take some time to appreciate the row of Georgian commercial buildings standing at Fulton and

Front streets. These brownstones with arched doors and wrought iron balconies made up a strikingly handsome block of stores when the seaport flourished. Look at the uneven roofline of the row. The mansard over 2 Fulton Street was added to increase the capacity of McKinley's Steamboat Hotel. At 92 South Street, part of the row, you'll find **Sloppy Louie's Restaurant,** unparalleled for bouillabaise and rude waiters.

If you're visiting the South Street Seaport in the summer, you may want to venture Sloppy Louie's or dine at the New Fulton Market and stay for the 7:30 or 8:00 P.M. concert on the pier. If not, catch a cab back to your hotel and choose from the list of accessible restaurants.

## TOUR 2

WHAT YOU'LL DO

* • Explore the Metropolitan Museum of Art (closed Mondays), perhaps joining a conducted tour, seeing a film, or browsing in gift shop.
 • Lunch at the Fountain museum cafe.
* • Visit to Guggenheim Museum (closed Mondays), with refreshments in cafe.
* • Visit to Cooper-Hewitt Museum (closed Mondays) and garden.
 • Self-tour and conducted tour of Lincoln Center, including dinner and performance.

HOW YOU'LL DO IT

• Cab from hotel to Metropolitan, Fifth Avenue at 82nd Street. Enter from 81st Street.
• Wheel six blocks from Metropolitan to Guggenheim, Fifth Avenue at 88th Street.
• Wheel three blocks from Guggenheim to Cooper-Hewitt, Fifth Avenue between 90th and 91st streets. Enter from 91st Street.

* Indicates restriction in time of visit.
$___/$___ indicates adult/child admission fees.
† All sites listed under "Restrooms" offer accessible facilities with wide stall doors and grab bars unless otherwise indicated.

- Cab from Cooper-Hewitt via Central Park to Lincoln Center, Broadway at 64th Street. Enter from 65th Street past first building.
- Cab from Lincoln Center to hotel.

THINGS TO KNOW

\* • Metropolitan Museum open daily except Mondays, 10:00 A.M. to 4:45 P.M. 'til 8:45 on Tuesday, Sunday 11:00 A.M.–4:45 P.M. Donation admission.
\* • Guggenheim Museum open daily, except Monday, 11:00 A.M. to 5:00 P.M., 'til 8:00 P.M. on Tuesday. Admission $1/50¢; Tuesdays free.
\* • Cooper-Hewitt Museum, open Wednesday–Saturday 10:00 A.M.–5:00 P.M.; Tuesday 10:00 A.M.–9:00 P.M.; Sunday 12:00 noon–5:00 P.M. Admission $1; Tuesdays free.
- Lincoln Center conducted tours 10:00 A.M. to 5:00 P.M. Admission $2.95/$1.75. Opera Cafe open daily 5:00 P.M. 'til end of intermission; Saturday noon–8:00 P.M. Grand Tier Restaurant open two hours before performance for ticket holders only during Met season. Reservations necessary. Top of the Met restaurant open 5:00 P.M. to 8:00 P.M.
- When ordering tickets by mail, address to proper theater box office, Lincoln Center, New York, N.Y. 10023, enclose self-addressed, stamped envelope. Specify "wheelchair location."

RESTROOMS †

- Metropolitan Museum, main floor
- Lincoln Center: Metropolitan Opera House, Avery Fisher Hall, New York State Theater, Alice Tully Hall, Vivian Beaumont Theater
- Jewish Museum, Fifth Avenue at 92nd Street (ramp plus 3 steps)

A day of palaces and mansions, of incomparable art treasures and quiet gardens, ending with the sound of music!

Begin with a cab ride to the neo-Renaissance palace that houses a million or more art treasures spanning fifty centuries. The **Metropolitan Museum of Art** is one of the great museums of the world, with dozens of exhibit halls devoted to everything from Greek and Roman art to Renaissance arms and European musical instruments. The Egyptian collection was opened in 1976 with 45,000 objects, one-third never on display before, making this the largest collection to be seen anywhere outside of Egypt. To be completed in 1978 will be the Temple of Dendur and in 1979, the Rockefeller and American wings.

Ask for a floor plan and choose from the wealth, including a look at the new Costume Institute and the superb museum shop. At lunch enjoy the sculpture and water at the **Fountain Restaurant,** or stop by the snack bar.

When you're ready to leave, wheel up Fifth Avenue. You'll come to several curb cuts and then for uninterrupted blocks you'll have easy rolling to the Guggenheim Museum and, when you continue, beyond to the Cooper-Hewitt Museum.

For most the controversial **Guggenheim** is a "must see." Architect Frank Lloyd Wright believed that architecture was the first art, making all others possible. He may have proved his point, as the art within seems secondary to the unique layout of the building. A one-quarter-mile-long ramp, with pictures hung alongside, curls around the three-story structure's interior. You can take an elevator to the second floor and there enjoy the one level room filled with modern masters' art. Then begin your descent and see how it goes. While in the museum, note the characteristic Wright details: the elevator decorations, the shape of the blue pond in the lobby, the motif on the gates outside.

At the **Cooper-Hewitt,** the new Smithsonian museum of design, you'll see more than exhibitions, for the collection is housed in one of Fifth Avenue's most fabulous mansions. Built by Andrew Carnegie in 1901, the neo-Georgian structure boasts the most lavish Victorian interior this side of a Louis Beebe railroad car. You'll find yourself right at home in the lush conservatory, the gilded rooms with massive chandeliers, the rich oak-paneled rooms, and the stunning hallway decked with tapestries. Explore the old garden, a remarkable enclave of azalea, rhododendron, wisteria, ivy, and old chestnut and apple trees as old as the house itself.

From the Cooper-Hewitt, take a cab to Lincoln Center via Central Park. This is a good time for a ten-minute tour; you might ask your driver to give you a brief ride around so you can take in the wealth of monuments, fountains, ponds, wooded paths, and flower beds. The Conservatory Lake is particularly charming, with its boaters and children sailing toy boats.

As a possible alternative, one block north of the Cooper-Hewitt is the **Jewish Museum,** housing the most extensive collection of Jewish ceremonial objects in the United States. The museum is in the mansion of banker Felix N. Warburg.

**Lincoln Center,** the $190 million, fourteen-acre cultural miniworld, has to be seen to be believed. The buildings are glorious, particularly the Metropolitan Opera House, with its two colorful Marc Chagall murals. Put yourself in the center of the plaza and enjoy the spectacle around you: Avery Fisher Hall (formerly Philharmonic Hall), the Eero Saarinen–designed Vivian Beaumont Theater, the New York State Theater, Alice Tully Hall, and the Library and Museum of the Performing Arts. Note also the outdoor sculpture pieces, including one by Henry Moore, and there's a leafy courtyard for rambling, as well as a reflecting pool and fountains.

Join the one-and-a-quarter-hour tour of the Center, during which you'll visit the Metropolitan Opera House for a look at the 24-carat gold ceiling. Dine at the outdoor cafe, in the **Opera Cafe,** the **Footlight Cafe,** the **Grand Tier Restaurant,** or **Top of the Met.** Explore the Library and Museum, with its headsets for music listening, its variety of exhibits.

Hopefully you'll have tickets in hand and will end your visit to Lincoln Center appropriately by attending a performance. In addition to experiencing the finest in theater, music, or dance, you'll see the Center as it was meant to be seen—chandeliers twinkling, lighted fountains splashing, and beautifully dressed people adding to the spectacle.

## TOUR 3

WHAT YOU'LL DO

- Breakfast at Rumplemayer's.
- Shop along Fifth Avenue.

$___/$___ indicates adult/child admission fees.
† All sites listed under "Restrooms" offer accessible facilities with wide stall doors and grab bars unless otherwise indicated.

- Lunch and tour the Museum of Modern Art.
- Visit St. Patrick's Cathedral.
- Tour Rockefeller Center, with ascent to the observation roof, dinner at the Promenade Cafe, film at Radio City Music Hall.
- Nightcap at Waldorf Astoria Hotel.

### HOW YOU'LL DO IT

- Cab from your hotel to Rumplemayer's at the St. Moritz Hotel, 59th Street and Fifth Avenue.
- Wheel two or three blocks along Fifth Avenue.
- Cab or push four blocks from Fifth Avenue at 57th Street to the Museum of Modern Art, 11 West 53rd Street.
- Wheel across the street from the Museum to Paley Park, Fifth Avenue and 53rd Street.
- Wheel two blocks from Paley Park to St. Patrick's Cathedral. Use 51st Street entrance.
- Wheel two blocks from St. Patrick's to Rockefeller Plaza, off Fifth Avenue between 50th and 49th streets.
- Cab from Rockefeller Center to Waldorf Astoria Hotel.
- Cab from Waldorf Astoria to your hotel.

### THINGS TO KNOW

- Rumplemayer's opens at 7:00 A.M. on weekdays, 8:00 A.M. on Sunday.
- Museum of Modern Art open Monday through Saturday 11:00 A.M.–6:00 P.M.; Thursday 11:00 A.M.–9:00 P.M.; Sunday noon–6:00 P.M. Admission $2/75¢. Tuesday free.
- St. Patrick's Cathedral open 6:00 A.M.–8:30 P.M.
- Rockefeller Center tour, 10:00 A.M.–5:00 P.M.. $1.80/$1.35. Observation Roof open 10:00 A.M.–9:00 P.M., April–September; 10:00 A.M.–7:00 P.M., October–March. $1.50/85¢.

### RESTROOMS †

- St. Moritz Hotel
- Saks Fifth Avenue, Fifth Avenue and 50th Stret.
- Museum of Modern Art (accessible, but doors less than 32 inches)

More sky-high views, fabulous art plus a sampling of Fifth Avenue's chic stores, and a journey back in time into the Art Deco 1930s at Rockefeller Center.

Begin with a cab ride to the fashionable hub, that point marked by the ornate Italian fountain where Fifth Avenue runs into Central Park. It's possible to get into the Plaza Hotel—the most famous of the landmarks at this juncture (which you do via the ballroom)—but instead sample a glamorous upstart, the St. Moritz Hotel and **Rumpelmayer's** cafe. You may choose to sit outside overlooking the park and from this vantage plan your day. By all means ramble across the street to the bookstalls, if they are in operation. Otherwise wheel past the Plaza and the fountain to the stores you've been hearing about most of your life. Among the choices within three blocks: the legendary **Tiffany & Co.,** where you can purchase an item for as little as $10 and have it wrapped as only Tif's can; **Godiva Chocolatier,** purveyor of perhaps the most sumptuous chocolates in the world; **Bergdorf Goodman,** with its Port of Call shop featuring treasures from exotic places; **Bonwit Teller,** featuring what you'd expect plus gourmet delights; **Ginori Fifth Avenue,** featuring Baccarat and St. Louis crystal; **Steuben Glass,** with the kinds of items on display that are sometimes chosen as gifts of state; and **F. A. O. Schwarz,** with toys for children of all ages. The General Motors Salon and Exhibit, with displays of automotive research and the latest GM cars is an interesting stop. There are several steps at the entrance, however.

With a little help from a friend, you can wheel your way four more blocks down Fifth Avenue and turn the corner at 53rd Street and the Museum of Modern Art—or have one of those polite clerks call a cab for you.

The **Museum of Modern Art,** devoted to the spectrum of modern art and design, including photography, film, pottery, furniture, graphic design, architecture, painting, and sculpture, is among the most sybaritic spots in town. Here you'll find a splendid outdoor sculpture garden, rich with Rodins and Calders, and some of the most delightful of the French impressionists, including Monet— huge canvases of his water lilies fill a portion of one room. To be enjoyed also are classic art films; your admission charge includes admission to the movie, but you have to reserve your theater ticket as soon as you arrive.

From the Museum wheel across Fifth Avenue to **Paley Park,** one of several "vest-pocket" parks dotting the city. Sit beneath the trees beside the waterfall and pretend you don't hear city traffic.

Next wheel two short blocks to **St. Patrick's Cathedral,** taking the zigzag ramp off Fifty-first Street into the edifice. Built in 1858, St. Patrick's is one of the finest Gothic structures in America.

Continue two blocks to Fifth Avenue and 50th Street and head for the Channel Gardens, lined with shops that lead to the glorious golden Prometheus statue with a curtain of fountains as backdrop. The building overlooking the statue is 30 **Rockefeller Center,** the RCA Building, one of the twenty-one buildings that make up this complex of skyscrapers. After a look at the gardens, head for this building.

A guided tour of the Center will show you some of this complex that covers twenty-four acres. You'll see some of the underground shops, the rooftop gardens, and take a look behind the scenes at the Radio City Music Hall. The tour leaves you on top of the world —literally. You'll know the tour is over when you are bid farewell on the seventieth-floor observation deck. You can take as long as you wish on the deck, asking questions of the guards and enjoying the view, which for some is more memorable than the one from the World Trade Center because of the view it affords of the Empire State Building. You can with little effort imagine King Kong climbing the chrome wonder and visualize those oldtime dirigibles mooring on the 120-foot mast that caps the building—the mast really was added for just that purpose!

While you're up in the air, stop for an avocado frappe at the lounge of the **Rainbow Room,** or return later.

If food is on your mind, take the elevator to the concourse level and the entrance to the **Promenade Cafe,** opening onto a huge patio that becomes an ice skating rink in the winter and an outdoor dining area in temperate weather. The menu includes such surprises as raspberry mousse, grasshopper pie, peach parfait, and, for those who look at items other than desserts, a fine selection of entrees including quiche and cioppino.

After dinner, visit the *grand dame* of New York hotels, the utterly opulent **Waldorf Astoria,** just down the street. You can with assistance ramble down the three blocks to the hotel. Otherwise hail or call a cab and end your day of New York glamor there in the most appropriate of lavish settings.

## TOUR 4

WHAT YOU'LL DO

- Ride tramway to Roosevelt Island.
* • Take bus ride around Roosevelt Island.
* • Visit United Nations for tour and lunch in Delegates' Dining Room (Monday through Friday).
- Visit Ford Foundation garden.
- Refreshments at new United Nations Plaza Hotel.
- Cruise around Manhattan on Circle Line sightseeing boat.
- Attend a performance at Carnegie Hall.
- Supper at the Russian Tea Room.

HOW YOU'LL DO IT

- Cab from hotel to Roosevelt Island tramway, Second Avenue at 60th Street.
- Cab from tramway to United Nations, First Avenue between 42nd and 48th streets.
- Wheel across street to Ford Foundation garden, First Avenue at 42nd Street.
- Wheel two blocks to United Nations Plaza Hotel, First Avenue at 44th Street.
- Cab from United Nations Plaza Hotel to Circle Line, Pier 83, end of West 43rd Street.
- Cab from Circle Line to Carnegie Hall, Seventh Avenue and 57th Street.
- Push a few doors to the Russian Tea Room, 150 West 57th Street.

THINGS TO KNOW

* • Roundtrip tramway ride to Roosevelt Island, $1. Wheelchair-accessible bus runs Wednesday, Saturday, Sunday 10:00 A.M.–noon, 4:00–7:00 P.M. Check times by calling 832–4540.

* Indicates restriction in time of visit.
$___/$___ indicates adult/child admission fees.

*  • United Nations tours begin about every ten minutes from
     9:15 A.M. to 4:45 P.M.; $2/$1 fee. Delegates' Dining Room
     open Monday through Friday; seating before 11:45 A.M. or
     after 2:00 P.M. Make reservation as soon as you arrive at the
     U.N.
   • Circle Line boats season is March–November, with sailings
     between 9:45 A.M. and 5:30 P.M. Three-hour tour $5/$2.50.
     Call 563–3200 re wheelchair-accessible restroom boats.
   • Obtain Carnegie Hall tickets via Ticketron or by mail, re-
     questing orchestra seats, since this is the only accessible area.
     Call the theater at 247–7459 to advise manager you are com-
     ing so he can have a house man available to operate the ele-
     vator that connects the entrance area with the orchestra tier.
   • Russian Tea Room serves after-theater supper from 9:30
     P.M.–1:00 A.M.

        RESTROOMS †

   • The United Nations, some Circle Line boats, and Carnegie
     Hall all offer accessible restrooms, but not necessarily with
     32-inch-wide stalls.

You'll get a bird's eye view of rooftop gardens as you soar over
Manhattan and then cross the East River to **Roosevelt Island** (formerly Welfare Island), now a model of innovative urban design.
In 1969 the state's Urban Development Corporation began to
transform the two-and-a-half-mile-long island into a complex of
mixed-income dwellings, schools, playgrounds, waterfront prome-
nades, and parks. Howard Logue, who masterminded New Haven's
successful urban renewal, created this New York "new community," with its buildings in human scale, its twisting Main Street,
and open spaces.

Since no cars, except those making deliveries, are permitted on
the island, the streets and walkways belong to the people—including wheelers. For among the residents of the new community are
those who formerly were patients at the Welfare Island hospitals.
Now many of the disabled live in specially designed housing that is
subsidized by the federal government. They can be seen in their
chairs, rolling along the streets, doing their shopping, and visiting
with their neighbors.

You'll see some of these happy islanders if you call ahead and request that a wheelchair-accessible minibus meet you at the tramway terminal. As you ride around the island, you'll also glimpse some of the seven buildings on the island that have been designated landmarks. One you won't miss is the 1889 Chapel of the Good Shepherd, now restored as a community center in the heart of town.

Even without the bus tour, you'll have the pleasure of the tramway ride and can get a close aerial look at what New Yorkers who live in "the Big Apple" call their "Little Apple."

Continue your day's adventure with a cab ride to the **United Nations.** Check with the information desk first thing to find out if any of the United Nations films are scheduled for the day, if there are any scheduled meetings you can attend, and to place your lunch reservation for the Delegates' Dining Room.

In the Delegates' Dining Room visitors are seated before 11:45 A.M. or after 2:00 P.M. as tables become available. As might be expected, the menu is international. Entrees, which range in price from $4.25 to $7, include such dishes as Boston sole, veal Parmigiana, and fresh pineapple with chicken salad. There's a featured unusual cocktail of the day, like a cherry blossom—a blend of cherry brandy, brandy, curacao, grenadine, and lemon juice.

You'll find a great deal to see on your own, including sculpture and art donated by member nations, murals designed by Fernand Leger, the dramatic Meditation Room, a space display featuring a chunk of moon rock, and stained glass panels by Marc Chagall. In the acres of parkland surrounding the buildings, you'll discover some 2,000 prize-winning rose bushes, 185 flowering cherry trees, 52 dwarf fruit trees, and a group of hawthorns, sweet gum, pin oaks, sycamores, and honey locust. With any luck, you'll share the garden with its views of the busy East River in the company of foreign delegates or U.N. staff members—perhaps a Burmese in a saffron robe, an Indian in a white dhoti, a Japanese with a briefcase and a camera, or an African in fancy headdress.

Take time for a look at the concourse-level United Nations post office. On the same level you'll find the United Nations Gift Center, the most cosmopolitan gift shop in New York City. Among the handicrafts from all over the world are wood carvings, jewelry, ethnic dolls, scarves, saris, brassware, and folk art.

While you're in the neighborhood consider making a stop at one of the modern architectural masterpieces in New York, the **Ford Foundation** building by Kevin Roche. The indoor garden is canopied by a 160-foot-high glass roof, giving the plant life hothouse impetus to grow. The results are lush. You'll find this a fragrant and inviting place to rest.

If you're ready for afternoon refreshments, you might stop by the stunning new **United Nations Plaza Hotel.** The Ambassador Grill, which you can reach by going down the elevator in the bank building that adjoins the hotel, gives one the feeling one has just crawled inside a multifaceted diamond. Ceilings of mirrored glass, prismatically reflecting and refracting light, are a marvel. You can have drinks here almost any time of day, or, sitting at a little table with a red rose in a bud vase, sample a tidbit from the pastry tray.

From the hotel you can go directly to the **Circle Line**'s Pier 83, hopefully in time to catch a late afternoon cruise around Manhattan Island. Your three-hour cruise will take you into the Upper Bay, where you'll see the Statue of Liberty, then along the East River back to the United Nations, followed by a jaunt on the Hudson River alongside Riverside Park, the Palisades of New Jersey, and the Cloisters and Fort Washington Park. Midtown towers come into view as you head back to the dock, and if the sun is setting, you'll see those concrete and steel skyscrapers melt into rosy hues. It's a beautiful time of day, and you couldn't be enjoying it from any better perspective. You can then cab back to midtown for a concert at **Carnegie Hall** and supper at the **Russian Tea Room**—or consider any one of a hundred other tantalizing combinations of sights and activities in this smorgasbord of a city.

## Other Accessible Attractions

Asia House Gallery, 112 East 64th Street
Bible House, 1865 Broadway at 61st Street
Caswell-Massey Pharmacy, Lexington Avenue at 48th Street
The Cloisters, Fort Tryon Park, 191st Street at Fort Washington Avenue (3 steps)
Daily News Building, 220 East 42nd Street
Jewish Museum, 1109 Fifth Avenue (3 steps)
Madison Square Garden Center, between Seventh and Eighth Avenue and 31st and 33rd streets

Merrill Lynch Investment Information Center, 165 Broadway
Mill at Burlington House, 1345 Sixth Avenue at 54th Street
Morris-Jumel Mansion, Roger Morris Park, West 160th Street
    at Edgecombe Avenue (3 steps)
Museum of Contemporary Crafts, 29 West 53rd Street
Museum of the American Indian, Broadway at 155th Street
    (use freight elevator)
Museum of the City of New York, Fifth Avenue at 105th
    Street (use 104th Street entrance)
Museum of Natural History, Central Park West at 79th Street
New York Public Library, Fifth Avenue at 42nd Street (use
    42nd Street entrance)
Pierpont Morgan Library, 29 East 36th Street (6 steps)
Planetarium, Central Park West at 81st Street (enter on 81st
    Street)
St. Bartholomew's Church, Park Avenue between 50th and
    51st streets
Temple Emanu-el, Fifth Avenue at 65th Street
Washington Square Park, south end of Fifth Avenue
Whitney Museum of American Art, 945 Madison Avenue at
    75th Street
Yeshiva University Museum, 2520 Amsterdam Avenue
Yankee Stadium, the Bronx

INTRODUCING

  *Rollin' On* adviser, wheeler Eileen Healy

*Title:* Office Manager, New York Easter Seal Society
*Telephone number:* (212) 532–8830
*Hometown:* New York
*Favorite tourist site:* Roosevelt Island as seen from the tramway
*Hidden corner:* the lighthouse on Roosevelt Island
*Rendezvous:* Mitchell's Place, First Avenue at 49th Street
*Offbeat restaurant:* Kitty Hawk's, 565 Third Avenue
*Place for music:* Lincoln Center
*View:* Battery Park
*Natural wonder:* Central Park
*Museum:* Metropolitan Museum of Art

*Ramble:* around the grounds of The Cloisters

*Non-tourist destination:* City Island in the northeast corner of the
Bronx

*Offbeat experience:* the Circle Line cruise around Manhattan

*Traditional restaurant:* Top of the Sixes, 666 5th Avenue

*Low-cost restaurant:* La Crepe, 57 West 56th Street

*Ice cream shop:* Rumpelmayer's at the St. Moritz Hotel

*Reading suggestion: This Is New York* by E. B. White

*Place to get a wheelchair repaired:* Check yellow pages under
Wheelchair Dealers for local listings.

*Tip on having a great time in New York:* Don't be afraid. There
is so much to enjoy. New Yorkers delight in being helpful.

# 8

# Philadelphia

There comes a moment. You round a corner to find a graceful iron gate inviting you to follow a red brick path into a recreated eighteenth-century garden where ivy carpets border beds of snapdragons, petunias, marigolds, and sweetpeas. You stop beneath the summerhouse shaded by hawthorn and mulberry, lost in the fragrance of lavender and thoughts of those people you know from the history books who enjoyed a similar garden on these same grounds over two hundred years ago. For you in this moment, the twentieth century of automobiles and airplanes is no more. You escape into the era of gaslights and horse-drawn carriages, into those years when brilliant minds devised a unique form of government and founded a nation. Travel, on occasion, moves us back into history. At times on such backward journeys our heart goes along on the expedition.

So it is in the old eighteenth-century city within the city of Philadelphia. Within the Independence National Historical Park, over forty blocks of streets and alleys, gardens and greenswards invite travelers to get lost in another century. Called the most historic mile in America, this urban historic park centered around Independence Hall boasts forty eighteenth-century homes, halls, banks, churches, libraries, and taverns—most open free of charge to anyone who calls.

In the 1940s a visitor to Philadelphia might have stopped for one hour to see the Liberty Bell and Independence Hall, if they could find their way through the jumble of warehouses surrounding the sites. Concerned citizens in 1948 finally got the federal government to create the Independence National Historical Park, and with the creation came $30 million in funds to tear down the dilapidated buildings that almost hid the famous monuments. Whole blocks were pulverized; historic buildings were restored and reconstructed. With surrounding buildings cleared away, the old historic structures came into view; after devoted scrubbing, the rosy hue of their brick exteriors also came into view.

This effort began Philadelphia's old city facelift, which was furthered when the government gave $100 million in matching funds to turn the city into a showplace of American history as the Bicentennial approached.

The result today after thirty years of effort is an old city that is brighter than it was two hundred years ago. The four blocks to the north of Independence Hall are now spacious parklands of green trees, benches, fountains, and pools. To the east of the Hall, a grassy park stretches three blocks, linking the historic core of the Park with the largest concentration of eighteenth-century buildings in existence in any city in the United States. Although some buildings are reconstructions like those in Williamsburg, most are original structures on their original sites.

For wheelchair travelers the Historical Park is a delight, with good curb cuts and enough accessible buildings to keep anyone busy for days. With its abundance of greenery, getting from one attraction to another is like going for a ramble in the park rather than down a city street.

And enjoying the out-of-doors and seeing the lovely old buildings and gardens is just a part. Consider what is inside these buildings. Exhibits bring history to life, and park service guides tell you in lively detail about the people who worked and lived in these structures when our nation was born. These knowledgeable interpreters open the way for many visitors to experience truly those historic days of our country's birth. So do the seven or more movies that are shown in various sites throughout the old city. The movies alone are worth a trip to Philadelphia. The quality of these films, most done for the Bicentennial celebration, is superb, and the overall impact after seeing several is surprising. By the time you're through, you'll have shared in Benjamin Franklin's home life, been with Thomas Jefferson as he wrote and rewrote the Declaration of Independence, joined the Congress as it nominated George Washington as the first president of the United States.

In addition to this eighteenth-century world, the old city of Philadelphia offers bright new twentieth-century buildings, built to harmonize with the low brick structures of the past. The city of Philadelphia, the state of Pennsylvania, and private companies offer a variety of sightseeing experiences, many put together for the Bicentennial. Among these are the multimedia Living History Museum; Penn Mutual Center, with its viewscopes and open-air observation terrace; and Penn's Landing, a renewed recreational center on the waterfront.

Beyond the old city are other sightseeing destinations, including the Victorian gingerbread City Hall, the new Chestnut Street Transitway shopping mall, and Fairmount Park, the largest city park in the world. In this 8000-acre woodland are nestled a host of sightseeing treasures, including the Memorial Hall from Philadelphia's 1876 Centennial Exposition, the oldest zoo in America, and ten historic mansions that go back to the 1770s.

Philadelphia is also a city of museums—over thirty, devoted to everything from science and medicine to the sculpture of Rodin and Afro-American art. Star of them all, of course, is the world-famous Philadelphia Museum of Art, a palace of medieval, French impressionist, and American art, plus period settings including a Hindu temple, a medieval chapel, and a Chinese scholar's study.

When it comes to life's more temporal pleasures, Philadelphia does all right. If you believe the old saw that summed up Philadelphia's one-time reputation at nightfall—"I went to Philadelphia and it was closed"—you're in for a surprise. Many a New York-bound theatrical play tries out in the five legitimate theaters here; nine little theaters and three summer theaters also offer a variety of productions. Cabarets and musical bars are easy to find, as are the free concerts, plays, and musical events held outdoors in the summer months.

Restaurants are scattered throughout this huge city of two million residents, with a good number concentrated in the city center and within and on the fringes of the old city. Because many restaurants are housed in old buildings, you cannot count on accessibility in Philadelphia, as you might in a newer city. This makes a list of accessible restaurants useful (see What You'll See and Do), to supplement that personal phone call asking those key accessibility questions.

## Planning Your Trip

Although summer does bring hot, humid days it's a tempting time to visit Philadelphia because of the unprecedented number of free concerts and other programs, particularly in the Independence National Historical Park area. To catch this summer fare, one might ideally plan on a visit in mid-June, when the programs have begun and the weather is still springlike. Otherwise spring or fall are your best bets, with spring favored because of the azalea blooms and cherry blossoms in Fairmount Park.

As for clothing, bring warm- and cool-weather trappings, including the usual sunburn preventatives. Since Philadelphia is a large, cosmopolitan city, you'll probably feel appropriately dressed if you're dressed for a city and not a resort.

To receive a packet of tourist information and a good city map, write to the Philadelphian Convention & Visitors Bureau, 1525 J. F. Kennedy Boulevard, Philadelphia, Pennsylvania 19102. Ask for information on the current package plans: combination hotel room and sightseeing and/or restaurant discount offerings.

If you don't have it already, write for the current *Guide to Philadelphia for the Handicapped*, available from the Mayor's Office for the Handicapped, Room 427, City Hall Annex, Philadelphia, Pennsylvania 19107; also request a copy of the current newsletter written for handicapped citizens and visitors.

## How to Get There

Philadelphia is served by Greyhound, Amtrak, and major airlines.

Greyhound brings you into the city at 17th and Market streets, ten blocks from the historic heart of old city Philadelphia.

Amtrak trains stop at the 30th Street Station. If a call is made in advance, a porter will meet you to assist you to the elevator that connects the track level with the main station. Otherwise you can find a porter after you disembark, or ask someone to call one for you. The station is close to the center of the city, about a $3 cab ride from the old city area. Restrooms are not accessible.

Philadelphia International Airport, located 6½ miles from the city center, is about an $8 cab ride from the Independence Mall area. The accessible airport includes restrooms that have been especially designed for wheelchair users. For a free brochure on the facilities for handicapped travelers, write to the City of Philadelphia, Division of Aviation, Philadelphia International Airport, Philadelphia, Pennsylvania 19153.

Cars with hand controls can be rented from Avis Rent a Car System in Philadelphia. (See Chapter 2 for car rental details.)

## Getting Around the City

As in any big city, driving in Philadelphia is a challenge and should be avoided at rush hour. By staying at a hotel in the old city area you can avoid a lot of that challenge, simply parking your car for two days near or in your hotel parking lot. On the third day of the itinerary suggested here, you'll be driving in the non-rush hour along Franklin Parkway to Fairmount Park. You can get a good map of the park by requesting one from the Fairmount Park Commission, Ohio House, Belmont Avenue and States Drive, Philadelphia, Pennsylvania 19131.

The Independence National Historical Park parking authority operates the least expensive garages in the old city—about $4 for a twenty-four-hour period. There's a lot at 6th and Market streets with entrances on 5th and 6th. Other lots are located at 801 Filbert Street and in center city at JFK Plaza, entrance on Arch Street.

As mentioned, self-pushing in the old city is relatively easy, with many curb cuts or very low curbs and wide brick walkways. The city is in the midst of a major program to increase the number of curb ramps, but until the job is completed you may need some assistance in getting around Society Hill and some of the areas outside the old city.

Accessibility is good in the old city, since most of the tourist attractions are federal buildings and non-government sites are up-to-date in design. At some of the National Park buildings you'll have to knock on the door and wait while a park service person lays down the ramp for you. At other times, as always, you'll simply have to know which entrance to head for.

As for restrooms, Philadelphia has a long way to go (in more ways than one!). Almost no restaurants offer accessible restrooms. Itineraries, therefore, have been planned around attractions that do have facilities and when possible are within only a few blocks of your hotel.

## Where to Stay

If you're coming to Philadelphia without a car you can get along very nicely in the old city using a few taxicabs and arm power. You'll be able to push to almost every major tourist site. If you want to see Fairmount Park and the Philadelphia Museum of Art, however, a car comes in handy, although you might also manage, and for less money, with a taxicab.

Within the Independence National Historical Park area is one ideally situated hotel, and that's all you really need if you plan far in advance so as to reserve one of the accessible guest rooms. It's the **Holiday Inn–Independence Mall** at 4th and Arch streets. Parking is on ground level with one step at the main entrance. The rooms are standard Holiday Inn, functional and unpretentious. What matters is the location and the pleasure you'll have pushing yourself at almost any hour to the surrounding parks and attractions. The 364-room hotel offers a swimming pool on the roof, free parking, a main dining room, a coffee shop, and the Blue Anchor Tavern.

Other accessible hotels offering special wheelchair rooms include:

Hilton Hotel, 34th and Civic Center Boulevard
Holiday Inn, 18th and Market streets
Holiday Inn, 36th and Chestnut streets
Holiday Inn, City Line Avenue
Holiday Inn, Airport
International House, 37th and Chestnut streets

Marriott, City Line Avenue
Penn Center Inn, 20th and Market streets
Sheraton Hotel, Airport

## What You'll See and Do

You'll see and do lots—maybe too much for some within the three days suggested here, but you can easily do a half day of suggested sightseeing and enjoy your swimming pool or sit under an elm tree on the Mall for the remainder of the day. The two days suggested here in the old city give you a look at the very best, most accessible attractions in the least amount of time. The third day requires driving your own car, renting one, or going by taxicab to the Philadelphia Museum of Art, the zoo and a brief ride through the park.

To find out what's going on around town, pick up a copy of *Where*, *Spotlight*, or the *Welcome Mat* newspaper—all free. If you have special questions or problems, call on *Rollin' On* adviser Bonnie Gellman at the Mayor's Office for the Handicapped; she's at (215) 686–7120.

When it comes to dining, you'll have a good number of choices, both in the old city and the nearby City Center area of Philadelphia.

### *Among the Accessible Restaurants*

Old City

Grendel's Lair, 500 South Street (one step)
Holiday Inn, 4th and Arch streets
Head House Tavern, 2nd and Pine streets
Lafayette House, 5th and Chestnut streets
Kite & Key Room, Benjamin Franklin Hotel, 9th and Chestnut streets
Old Original Bookbinder's, 125 Walnut Street (enter via "exit" door)
Penn's Welcome, Penn Mutual Tower
Riverfront Restaurant, Delaware and Poplar streets
Sugar Cone, 414 South 2nd Street

Wicker Basket, Penn Mutual Tower
Wildflowers, 516 South 5th Street

Center City

Bains, 215 South Broad Street
Gallery Mall, 9th and Market streets (restaurants include the
    Market Fair, Magic Pan, Sbarro's, Open Hearth)
Happy Gardens, 134 North 10th Street (one step)
House of Mignon, 1614 Ludlow Street
Kelly's, 1620 Ludlow Street (one step)
La Crepe, 1425 Chestnut Street
La Diet, 1634 Ludlow Street (one step)
Ralphy's, 760 South 9th Street (one step)
Stouffer's Restaurant, 1526 Chestnut Street
Tarello's, 1623 Chestnut Street
Wanamaker's Lunch Room, 13th and Market streets
Winston's, 15th and Locust streets
Zum-Zum, 1527 Chestnut Street (use side entrance)

Other Locations

Asia, 4746 North Broad Street
Doc Watson's, 39th and Sansom streets
Dragon Gate, 913 Race Street
Fisher's, 3545 North Broad Street (one step)
Franklin Stove, 555 City Line (one step)
House of Pagano's, 3633 Walnut Street
Kum Lim, 2417 Welsh Road (one step)
Lotus Inn, 1010 Race Street
Magic Pan, City Line Avenue at Decker Square
Open Hearth, City Line and Belmont Avenue
Red Lobster, Roosevelt Boulevard at Walsh
Rustler's Steak House, Roosevelt and Robbins Avenue
Seafood Shanty, Roosevelt Boulevard at Cottman Street
2601 Parkway Restaurant, 26th and Parkway
Valle's Steak House, 9495 Roosevelt Boulevard

## TOUR 1

WHAT YOU'LL DO

- Tour Independence Hall, Congress Hall, Old City Hall, and the Liberty Bell Pavilion.
- Visit the Penn Mutual Center observation roof and exhibit.
- Lunch at the Wicker Basket.
- Visit the Atwater-Kent Museum.
* • Tour the Living History Center (closed Mondays), view film, have refreshments in Center's garden cafe.
- Dine at hotel, Lotus Inn, or Penn's Welcome.
* • See the sound and light spectacle at Independence Hall (summer only).

HOW YOU'LL DO IT

- Push two-and-a-half blocks to Independence Mall, Market and Walnut streets between 5th and 6th streets.
- Push one block to Penn Mutual Center, 6th and Walnut streets.
- Push two-and-a-half blocks to Atwater-Kent Museum, 15 South 7th Street (enter thru garden).
- Push two blocks to Living History Center, 6th and Race streets.
- Cab to hotel, to Lotus Inn, or Penn Mutual Center.
- Cab or push two-and-a-half blocks to Independence Mall.
- Cab or push from Independence Mall three blocks back to your hotel.

THINGS TO KNOW

- Independence National Historical Park buildings open 9:00 A.M.–5:00 P.M.
- Penn Mutual Center observation roof and exhibits open 10:00 A.M.–5:00 P.M. Admission $1.40/90¢.

---

\* Indicates restriction in time of visit.

$___/$___ indicates adult/child admission fees.

† All sites listed under "Restrooms" offer accessible facilities with wide stall doors and grab bars unless otherwise indicated.

- Atwater-Kent Museum open 8:30 A.M.–4.30 P.M. Free admission.
* • Living History Center open 9:30 A.M.–6:00 P.M. Tuesday–Thursday and Saturday; Friday 9:30 A.M.–8:00 P.M.; Sunday 12:30–6:00 P.M. Film shown on the hour. Admission $3.50/$2; half price Friday after 5:00 P.M.
* • Sound and light spectacle at 9:00 P.M. Free. Summer only.

RESTROOMS †

- Penn Mutual Tower
- Living History Center

After breakfast at your hotel, push two blocks to Market and Fifth streets, where you'll see the handsome **Liberty Bell Pavilion.** You'll hear the taped story of how the bell was moved from the State House tower as the British approached Philadelphia, hidden in an Allentown church, and how it cracked while tolling for the funeral procession of Chief Justice John Marshall. Note how the bell is silhouetted against Independence Hall, a sight to be seen any time of day or at night when the Pavilion is lighted.

Head towards **Independence Hall,** making a stop for tourist literature and information at the Visitors' Center kiosk at Chestnut and 5th streets. Look for brochures that offer discounts on the admission to such sites as Penn Mutual Center, the Living History Center, and the Philadelphia Museum of Art.

There's a curb cut at 6th and Chestnut streets, so you may want to go that route to Independence Hall. Once at the Hall, enter or knock on the side door for a conducted tour of the building that began as a provincial government building and became the birthplace of a new nation. You'll see the Assembly Room where delegates from each of the thirteen colonies sat at assigned tables. Note the inkstand on the president's desk, actually used by the delegates to sign both the Declaration of Independence and the Constitution. Across the hall you'll see the Supreme Court chambers.

Next visit the twin **Congress Hall** and **Old City Hall,** on opposite sides of Independence Hall. Used as the United States capitol while the permanent capitol was being built in Washington, D.C.,

Congress Hall was the site for the inauguration of George Washington and John Adams. Old City Hall, which reopened after restoration work in 1975, was the site where the U.S. Supreme Court heard its first cases. In these buildings also you'll hear from a park interpreter who also will answer your questions. Be sure to look for the refreshment table in Congress Hall where delegates got their sips of grog, and note the eighteenth-century poster display as you enter Old City Hall.

From under shady trees outside you'll want to stop to appreciate the beauty of these Georgian buildings. If it's summer you may be lucky and run into a fife and drum corps playing "Yankee Doodle Dandy." This is the spot where you'll be coming back later in the day to enjoy the famous sound and light spectacle.

Your next stop can be **Penn Mutual Tower,** set in a direct line with Independence Hall on Walnut between 6th and 5th streets. Take the glass elevator to the twenty-second-floor view tower, which opened in 1976. As you ascend you'll get a breathtaking view of the whole Independence National Historical Park area, a vista that can be leisurely enjoyed once you've arrived at the towertop observation area and exhibit. There's a steep ramped incline as you roll out from the elevator, but one of the hostesses stationed at the elevator will be there to give you a hand if need be.

You'll have a lot to see and do here: two movies, seven museum exhibit areas, an outdoor observation deck, and walls of windows with audiovisual explanations. You'll take a visual tour of a city with abundant greenery, the blue Delaware River lively with cargo vessels and even an anchored masted ship with white sails fluttering, fascinating rooftops that are brown, red, pale green, and cupola-decked. As you wait for the movies to begin, you'll have time to study the exhibits, noting such charming items as a 1700-vintage beaver bonnet, Episcopal silver shoe buckles (Quakers didn't wear silver buckles), an 1885 friendship quilt, clay pipes excavated from Society Hill, and a busybody mirror—the gadget eighteenth- and nineteenth-century folks fastened outside their windows to better see what was happening up and down the street.

For lunch you can choose between two restaurants in the Penn Mutual Building, the **Penn's Welcome** and the casual **Wicker Basket,** serving twenty-five varieties of hot and cold sandwiches.

To reach either, descend from the tower to the street and roll into the next-door Penn Mutual Building. A receptionist will indicate where the rear service elevators are that will take you to the two restaurants. As an alternate, you can buy hot dogs, ice cream, soda, and other portables from the street vendors around the Mall and lunch outdoors or, for the energetic, push up Chestnut Street to the numerous bakeries, cafes, and coffee shops to be found in this newly renovated shopping area that runs between 6th and 18th streets.

After lunch push two-and-a-half blocks from Penn Mutual to the **Atwater-Kent Museum** at 15 South 7th Street, entering from the garden. Once the site for the Franklin Institute, the lovely 1825 marble edifice is set in a green garden complete with a historic guardhouse. Inside you'll see some remarkable treasures: old carousel animals, including an 1840s-vintage wooden pig built for two; a lottery ticket to raise money for the 1776 Congress; a seventeenth-century clock with French soldiers marching and tooting horns on the hour; an electric Pope Waverly battery-charged car; and a wooden cigar store "gentleman" with dundreary whiskers (most of these kinds of models were Indians, you recall). In addition you'll see several fine dioramas, a model of Elfreth Alley, a toy shop with everything from Christmas tree ornaments to pedlar dolls, plus a recreation of the first bank founded in North America, complete with scales, ledgers, and fire buckets.

Across the street from the Atwater-Kent Museum is the **Balch Institute,** another 1976 addition, featuring the ethnic history of America. Included among the displays are dolls from fifty nations, a display of keepsakes brought by immigrants on their passage to the New World, and a glory of hand-made banners that express in fabric scenes—such as Dutch appliqued children ice skating on a blue satin lake—the heritage of America's many cultures. The banners, set in a room with soundscopes on which one hears immigrants speaking about America, are works of art all done by local high school youngsters.

Next door is the **Graff House,** administered by the National Park Service. This is the site where Thomas Jefferson drafted the Declaration of Independence. Only the first-floor exhibit area is accessible, but you will see Jefferson's original draft of the Declaration of

Independence with the clause renouncing slavery, which was deleted when the document was ratified. Also to be seen is a seven-minute film on Jefferson's contribution to our history.

Time for an Italian ice or other refreshment from one of those sidewalk vendors? If so, you'll find several nice gardens, including the one behind the Atwater-Kent Museum, for a rest.

When the spirit moves you, continue your sightseeing by pushing up 7th Street to Market and then along 6th, heading north two blocks to the **Living History Center** at 6th and Race streets. This new $11.5 million museum was designed to convey the total American experience since 1776 through film and advanced multimedia technology. The effect is something like a three-ring circus. There are twenty-eight displays depicting the American past, present, and future in the 16,000 square feet of exhibit space, and everything is going on at once! Among the things to discover: an overhead screen flashing a continuous series of the best known American symbols; a sixty-four-screen slide presentation called "To the New World," showing the impact immigration has had on America; a history walk (or roll) presenting a chronological survey of American history from Columbus's landing to the present; Future Theater, a film project portraying America as a nation of planners, with a bank of voting machines where visitors can cast their ballots on what they think the nation's priorities should be; the Quiz Machine, a computer that flashes questions about U.S. history on a screen, together with multiple choice answers; the birthday machine, which offers a print-out of historic events that happened on the day that the visitor punches in; a series of fifty audience-activated audio shows, heard through stereophonic headsets, dealing with historic moments in American history—and more.

Two films are included in the price of admission: one the fifteen-minute *To Secure These Rights* production about a young boy who takes a journey back into history; and *American Years*, shown on a seven-story-high IMAX theater screen. This forty-eight-minute film is by Academy Award–winner Francis Thompson, creator of the New York World's Fair winner *To Be Alive*.

Don't miss the rooftop "Historytoy" playground with its giant replicas of early American toys that move when children swing, spin, or seesaw. Beneath the rooftop playground is a cafe that opens onto a courtyard enhanced by a waterfall and shaded by young trees. This is a good spot for refreshment and people-watching, but don't plan on dinner, as the food service stops at 5:00 P.M.

When it's time for dinner, you are about three blocks from the Holiday Inn and four blocks from one of the best accessible Chinese restaurants in town, the **Lotus Inn** at 1010 Race Street.

Whether you dine at your hotel and include time for a rest or swim, or push or cab to the Lotus Inn, plan your time so that you can be at Independence Hall at 9:00 P.M. for the sound and light spectacle. The fifty-minute presentation, titled "The American Bell," uses the dramatic technique developed in France over thirty years ago for recreating historic events on the sites where they actually occurred. In this, the first application of the sound and light technique in the western hemisphere, an invisible cast moves inside the Hall as lighting effects are seen both inside and outside the building. Perhaps the only way to think about the spectacle is to think back on how it used to be listening to radio drama and seeing the visions the mind's eye conjured up. It is the same with the sound and light spectacle, for much is left to the imagination.

With visions of the Pennsylvanian colonists working frantically to remove the bell from the tower before the British arrive, you may want to stop for an evening look at the Liberty Bell as you wheel back to the hotel. If you do, you end your day of sightseeing where it began, but as you look at the bell in the evening, it may have new meaning for you.

## TOUR 2

WHAT YOU'LL DO

- Tour U.S. Mint.
- Tour Friends' Meeting House.
- Join conducted tour of the Second Bank.
- Lunch in the Tea Garden.
- Visit the Visitors' Center, view film.
- Visit the Franklin Court museum.
- Tour Society Hill, with stop at Perelman Antique Toy Mu-

† All sites listed under "Restrooms" offer accessible facilities with wide stall doors and grab bars unless otherwise indicated.

seum, New Market shopping complex, Head House Square, and libations at Head House Tavern.

- Dinner at Old Original Bookbinder's Restaurant.

HOW YOU'LL DO IT

- Push one block to U.S. Mint, 5th and Arch streets.
- Push one block to Friends' Meeting House, 4th and Arch streets (enter east side door).
- Push three blocks to Second Bank of the United States, 421 Chestnut Street (enter east door).
- Push one block to Visitors' Center, 3rd and Chestnut.
- Push one-and-a-half blocks to Franklin Court, Oriana Street between Market and Chestnut streets.
- Cab from Franklin Court to Perelman Antique Toy Museum, 270 South 2nd Street.
- Push three blocks to Head House Tavern and Square, 2nd and Pine streets.
- Cab from Head House Tavern to hotel or directly to Old Original Bookbinder's Restaurant, 2nd and Walnut streets.
- Cab from Bookbinder's via Penn's Landing back to hotel.

THINGS TO KNOW

- U.S. Mint open 9:00 A.M.–3:30 P.M. Admission free.
- Friends' Meeting House open 10:00 A.M.–4:00 P.M. Free admission.
- Second Bank open 9:00 A.M.–5:00 P.M. Free.
- Carryout lunch available at Lafayette Cafe, 5th and Chestnut streets. Tea Garden serves snacks.
- Visitors' Center open 9:00 A.M.–5:00 P.M. Free.
- Franklin Court open 9:00 A.M.–5:00 P.M. Free.
- Perelman Antique Toy Museum open 9:30 A.M.–5:00 P.M. Admission $1.
- Bookbinders' open 11:30 A.M. weekdays, noon Saturday, 1:00 P.M. Sunday.

RESTROOMS †

- U.S. Mint
- Second Bank of the United States
- Visitors' Center

During its days of glory when our new nation was being forged, Philadelphia was the intellectual, political, and commercial center of the New World. As you continue your journey back into the eighteenth and nineteenth centuries during your second day in Philadelphia, you'll see the meeting places, commercial institutions, homes, and taverns that turn those facts in history books into living reality.

Begin just a few doors from your hotel with a visit to the **Friends' Meeting House,** which is on the site where Penn's colony of Quakers first met, working out the practical details of his revolutionary "holy experiment." Here you'll see the original hand-hewn benches, made from trees cut down to clear the land, and an exhibit of period clothing, Bibles, and farm and household items. The dioramas of William Penn give a memorable account of the founding of his New World province based on his belief that men could live together in peace and freedom regardless of their religious beliefs.

As you roll on to the **U.S. Mint** one block west, look inside the gate at the **Christ Church Burial Ground** at the corner of 5th and Arch streets to see the Benjamin Franklin grave. Across the street, note the Free Quaker Meeting House (inaccessible), restored to look as it did when a faction of Quakers broke away from the main pacifist body to fight in the Revolutionary War.

Enter the Mint via the ramp on the northern side of the building. Originally a small cluster of brick buildings when it began turning out coins in 1792, the U.S. Mint was the first public building erected by the government. Now the facility covers three city blocks and is capable of producing over 1.5 million coins per hour.

You can take a self-guided tour along a gallery with windows that look down on the various operations in coin-making. Signs identify each process and a taped explanation at each station fills you in on what is happening below. Most fascinating perhaps is the rolling out of the melted metal from 6-inch-thick, 9-foot-long blocks to coils that are 109 feet long and .05 inch thick. Visit also the Relic Room to see a historic collection of coins and to see the bronze medals and proof sets on sale at the shop.

Continue your sightseeing by following 4th Street to Chestnut Street and the **Second Bank of the United States,** during its heyday one of the most influential financial institutions in the world. Built in 1819, the building is a partial imitation of the Parthenon and an outstanding example of Greek Revival architecture. Inside in the main lobby you'll see the delicately shaded half-barrel Roman-style ceiling, cast iron safe doors painted to look like wood, and the original clock—still running. Explore the first- and second-floor galleries filled with almost one hundred Charles Wilson Peale paintings. Of particular interest is the Washington Gallery, with its carved pine sculpture of Washington by William Rush, the Peale painting of Martha, a silhouette, and a Pennsylvania German *fraktur* print.

The Foreign Dignitary Room, furnished in articles from the Empire period, is graced by a Waterford crystal chandelier that once hung in Independence Hall. Don't miss the second-floor gallery of early portraits of artists and scientists, including Noah Webster, and the Pennsylvania Gallery of pre- and post-Revolutionary War paintings of Philadelphians.

Right beside the Second Bank is the **Tea Garden,** which serves sandwiches and soft drinks, including squash, a colonial concoction. You can lunch in the garden setting or pick up some edibles from Lafayette House at 5th and Chestnut streets.

From the Tea Garden a number of paths crisscross this beautifully maintained National Park area. With a little wheeling you can see the oldest bank building in America, the First Bank of the United States, on what was known as Treasury Row, 3rd Street between Chestnut and Walnut streets; the architectural masterpiece of the park, the semicircular Philadelphia Exchange; the recreated eighteenth-century garden maintained by the Pennsylvania Horticultural Society at 325 Walnut Street; the magnolia garden and rose garden on Walnut between 4th and 5th streets; Carpenters Hall, across the street from the Tea Garden; and **City Tavern** at 2nd and Walnut streets. Although the Tavern, which opened recently after reconstruction in 1975, is not generally accessible, you can have lunch served to you by costumed barmaids in the garden or in the first-floor dining room, which is accessible via the kitchen. If you're a history nut with sauteed breast of capon with ham and sherried cream sauce on your mind—or a fruit and cheese plate, Indian pudding, cyder shrub, or English trifle—you may find the experience of dining in this "most genteel of meeting places" worth a phone call and a little trouble.

After lunch and a rolling tour, drop in at the **Visitors' Center** for a rest while watching the free movie *Independence,* produced by 20th Century Fox and starring Eli Wallach.

Afterwards push on to **Franklin Court,** entering on Oriana Street off Chestnut between 3rd and 4th streets. Since historians were unable to provide enough detail for a legitimate reconstruction, only a steel frame marks the original space where Franklin's house stood. What is there, however, is a $6 million underground museum reached by ramp. Within this subterranean museum you'll see an exhibit of Frankliniana, including an original Franklin stove, his desk, and his carriage. Passing through the Hall of Mirrors, where you see in neon lights the words that describe Franklin's diverse abilities, you enter a large room with a number of exhibits, including the Franklin Exchange. You dial a number on a telephone and hear comments from such famous men as John Keats, Woodrow Wilson, and John Adams about Franklin. There's an exhibit of Franklin quotes, a moving model called Franklin on the World Stage, and a fine movie that lets you in on Franklin's domestic life.

Above ground again, enjoy the garden of mulberry and plane trees and take a peek inside the eighteenth-century post office, the business office of the *Aurora* newspaper, a print shop, and other small houses. (As you leave Oriana Street, you may want to stop by the Maritime Museum, with paintings relating to the sea, charts, navigational instruments, scrimshaw, weapons, scale models, and whaling harpoons.)

From Franklin Court you can go by cab (or wheel three longish blocks) to **Society Hill,** one of the nation's best known and most successful urban renewal and historical restorations. You'll see more authentic buildings standing on their original foundations in this twenty-five-square-block area than in any other city in the United States.

Begin with a visit to Philadelphia's tallest colonial restoration, the Abercrombe House, now housing the **Perelman Antique Toy Museum.** Here is the largest collection of antique toys in the world —there are over 2000 on display. Although you won't be able to play with them yourself, the curator sometimes winds up or otherwise demonstrates the mechanical actions of the fire engines, stage coaches, hansom cabs, and all manner of waving and wagging animals. Among the treasures: an animated bank that is an elephant tossing pennies into its slotted back, a cap pistol with figures of men and animals that kick, buck, or bite when the cap is exploded, and an automaton of Ulysses S. Grant smoking a cigar.

Across the street from the Toy Museum, note the Man Full of Trouble Tavern (inaccessible), the only Philadelphia tavern remaining from colonial times. Then push along 2nd Street for two interesting blocks to the **Head House** meeting place, with its covered arcade for tradesmen stretching behind. Today artists show their wares on summer weekends. Although the street is very bumpy, you may find it wheelable. From this central location you have a number of sightseeing options, all within two blocks. First you can stop at the famous **Head House Tavern** (one steep step). This colonial-style restaurant serves period fare as well as some of the more modern favorites—including libations. Just around the corner at Stamper Blackwell Court on Pine Street, you can explore a typical restored courtyard, this one with lamps, neat brick walkways, shady trees, borders of flowers, and the charming Mustang sculpture.

Two blocks away is the modern **New Market** complex, which won a 1963 HUD design award. By being assisted up a very steep ramp you can see Water Plaza, a wood and water sculpture that includes a waterfall and large reflecting pool. A number of shops and restaurants are level, including an outdoor cafe, toy shop, and stationery and jewelry boutiques. If you can negotiate three high steps, you'll find a good portion of the complex accessible, for beyond the old bake house is an accessible elevator that will take you to the other two levels, including the one that opens onto the outdoor courtyard of the Ristorante Focolare. There's also an accessible indoor restaurant portion.

At the corner of Lombard and 2nd streets, you'll come upon an open plaza where on summer evenings you'll hear local musicians. This is the ideal spot to take in all the local scene—the people and the color and texture of the varied architecture: the pale peach, orange, and rust hues of the renovated brick structures; the white pointed roofs capping the stalls, the pale green dome of a church, the towering wall of apartment houses, the banners fluttering from standards in front of stores and restaurants, the reproduction gas street lamps.

From the plaza, it's six or seven blocks to **Bookbinder's** at 2nd and Walnut streets, so hail or call a cab. When your cabbie lets you out, notice if he gets out himself to enjoy the free cup of coffee offered from a sidewalk urn by the management of Bookbinder's.

Enter via the exit door and enjoy this Philadelphia institution, which opened its doors in 1865. You'll choose from an extensive menu of fresh fish, including Columbia River salmon, fresh scrod, and swordfish in anchovy sauce—in season. If you want to dine lightly, you could go the clam chowder or snapper soup route with French bread and finish off with cheesecake or walnut and apple pie.

After dinner you may want to return to your hotel via Penn Landing, one of the city's newest historic renovations. A number of historic vessels, including Harry Truman's yacht and the old cargo vessel the **Moshulu,** now a restaurant, can be seen. From the Landing, **Rainbow Boat Tours** operates two-hour cruises that go fourteen miles to the mouth of the Schuylkill River. The upper deck is accessible to wheelchair users. Tours depart at 11:00 A.M., 1:30 P.M. and 7:00 P.M. daily.

## TOUR 3

WHAT YOU'LL DO

- Visit the Philadelphia Museum of Art.
- Lunch at the Water Works Cafe.
- Tour Fairmount Park.
- Visit the Philadelphia Zoo.
- Dine at the Belmont Mansion.
- Attend a performance at the Playhouse in the Park.

HOW YOU'LL DO IT

- Drive to the Museum of Art, 26th Street and Franklin Parkway.
- Drive behind the Museum to the Water Works Cafe.
- Drive through Fairmount Park via Sedgley Drive, East River

---

$___/$___ indicates adult/child admission fees.
† All sites listed under "Restrooms" offer accessible facilities with wide stall doors and grab bars unless otherwise indicated.

Drive, Girard Avenue Bridge, 34th Street, South Concourse
Drive, Belmont Drive.

- Push across the way from the Belmont Mansion to the Playhouse in the Park.
- Drive from the Playhouse via West River Drive and the Parkway to your hotel.

### THINGS TO KNOW

- Museum of Art open 9:00 A.M.–5:30 P.M. Admission $1.50/
75¢; free Sundays. Tours 10:00 A.M.–3:00 P.M. on the hour.
- Water Works Cafe open 11:00 A.M.–6:30 P.M. daily.
- Zoo open 9:30 A.M.–5:00 P.M. daily. Admission $2.50/$1.
Storybook key to audio information, 60¢.
- Belmont Mansion serves dinners 5:00 P.M.–8:00 P.M., from
4:00 P.M. on Saturday. Reservations advised.
- Playhouse in the Park open June–August nightly. Call GR7–
1700 for ticket information.

### RESTROOMS †

- Museum of Art
- Zoo
- Playhouse in the Park

A day for discovering Philadelphia's treasury of art works and
for exploring one of the most beautiful recreational complexes in
the country. This is a day of superlatives, when you'll see what
some say is America's most beautiful building and the world's
largest city park.

Begin with a drive down Philadelphia's Champs Elysées, the
Benjamin Franklin Parkway. This tree-lined boulevard, cut in
1926, links City Hall and the Philadelphia Museum of Art. On
either side of the Parkway are the city's wealth of institutions: the
Franklin Institute, the Free Library, Moore College of Art, the
Academy of Natural Science, the Cathedral of St. Peter and Paul,
and the Rodin Museum.

The Rodin Museum may be accessible by the time you get there,
via a new rear entrance. If so, you can see the sunlit gallery, with
its casts, watercolors, and drawings by the famous French artist.

The entrance portal is a reproduction of part of the one at the ancient Chateau d'Issy; the building is of French Renaissance design. The garden of quiet pools and flowers is an unofficial bird sanctuary.

Proceed up the Parkway to the **Philadelphia Museum of Art,** circling the Leif Ericson Memorial Fountain and the elaborate Washington Monument, with its menagerie of animals—bison, bears, and moose. The pools at the base represent the four great waterways of America.

The Museum of Art, built for the great Centennial Exposition held in Philadelphia in 1876, may be the most beautiful building in America, particularly as seen at night when floodlit. The mountain of stairs at the front entrance was made even more famous by the *Rocky* movie, and today they're used in the early mornings by the new breed of joggers who were influenced by that movie.

The ten acres of monument seem even larger from within. The Great State Hall is awesome and dramatically suited to the thirteen tapestries and "Diana" sculpture at the top of the stairway. Within this treasure house of a half million works of art, you'll find early Italian religious art; works from England, Holland, France; American rooms installed intact; pre-Columbian and modern art; Pennsylvania Dutch folk art; a medieval chapel; a Roman fountain and courtyard; a Japanese tea house and garden; a Chinese scholar's study; and a Hindu temple. The museum is known for its period rooms; it was one of the first to display furniture with appropriate art objects, thus creating a total period environment.

Notable among the many exhibits is the newly opened American wing. The exhibit encompasses the total American experience and includes a Pennsylvania Dutch room, where one sees the daily household items of these early settlers. Among these is a shiny red clay sugar bowl, a *sgraffito*-decorated toolbox, a meat fork and spatula, a trick box, wooden butter print-maker, decorated eggs, a walnut armchair, a wardrobe inlaid with sulphur paste and brass, and a 1780-vintage pin cushion stand. The Shaker room shows a period bedroom plus such personal and household objects as a hickory-and-pine bucket, maple rocking chair, desk of bird's-eye maple, a padded taffeta bonnet, denim shoes, a spectacle case, comb cleaner, clothespin, and tongue depressor.

Of course you could spend days, but with the tour you'll see the highlights, and on your own you can explore your particular favorites. The museum shop is one of the best of its kind, with jewelry, reproductions, books, and prints.

You can lunch at the quite unmemorable museum cafeteria or enjoy the sunlight and view from the Water Works Cafe, which lies behind the Museum on Aquarium Drive. From the Museum, follow East River Drive to the Lincoln Monument, circle the monument, and take Aquarium Drive.

The **Water Works Cafe** is part of the Fairmount Water Works, a romantic callection of buildings built between 1819 and 1822. From the outdoor porch of the cafe, you overlook an extravaganza of classical temples in a waterland of pools, waterfalls, a dam, and river. This is also a good site for seeing Boathouse Row and the scullers crewing on the river as their coach shouts instructions from a motor boat.

The Cafe serves an imaginative selection of sandwiches, salads, and desserts, including a fresh and dried fruit salad featuring nuts, grated coconut, and ricotta cheese. And don't miss the hazelnut cheesecake!

From the Cafe you can continue your drive, viewing some of the major park sites from your car window and even getting out and going in to see others. A good route is to retrace your course back to the Lincoln Monument, then left at the first road you reach, which is Lemon Hill Drive. See the Lemon Hill House, which was built by Robert Morris, a signer of the Declaration of Independence and financier of the Revolution. Continue right on Lemon Hill Drive to the Gazebo and Grant's Cabin, occupied by the general as headquarters. Retrace your path back to East River Drive and follow it to the Girard Avenue Bridge.

Crossing the bridge, turn left onto 34th Street, and you'll be at the entrance to the **Philadelphia Zoo,** another remainder of the 1876 Centennial Exposition. Along the almost totally accessible forty-two acres that shelter 1600 animals, you'll see a lovely collection of old trees: Japanese cherry, elm, sugar maple, copper beach, and ginkgo. Also noteworthy are the statues of animals, including a lion rescuing a lamb from a pack of wolves.

Perhaps the most idyllic spot is the large pond that a dozen or more varieties of swan, geese, and ducks call home. It's the very pond where E. B. White's creations, Louis and Serena, met as told in his story "The Trumpet of the Swan."

If historic houses interest you, the 1771 **Solitude House,** which served as the Zoo's first office, is a must. The Zoo evolved around the house, inhabited by an eccentric bachelor who took to feeding the wild bear and deer that came to his grounds. Although the top floors are not accessible, you can see the hallway with its fine wrought iron stairway and the parlor with its Sheridan bookcases and decorated ceiling. If you think the house was elegant for its time, you're right; Solitude House was the first home in America to be insured by Lloyds of London.

Another historic house is across the street from the Zoo. It's the Letita Street House, restored by the city of Philadelphia in 1976 and opened as an historic house museum.

If you follow 34th Street, it will become South Concourse Drive and will pass the Sweetbriar House, which stands now exactly as it did in 1797. At the top of the hill is the Smith Memorial, an indoor playground with a sliding board ten children wide, an outdoor swimming pool, gardens, and even a kitchen. Pass between the two spires to reach the glass-domed Memorial Hall, the only major building remaining from the Centennial Exposition. Near it you'll see the beautifully reconstructed seventeenth-century Japanese scholar's house, a tea house, and garden. The Horticultural Gardens are adjacent, and Belmont Drive connects with the gardens, your next route. Follow the drive to Belmont Plateau for a sweeping panorama of the river and city skyline. The rambling **Belmont Mansion** with its outdoor terrace is the closest thing to a country inn within city limits. You'll feel as if you're on a vacation in the country, the country of a century ago.

At the **Playhouse in the Park** you can see some of the best little theater around. The Playhouse is the home of the Philadelphia Actors Theater and also offers occasional Broadway try-outs.

After a memorable evening of dinner and theater, follow Belmont Mansion Drive back toward the Horticultural Gardens area, but just before reaching it turn left onto Montgomery Drive. Follow Montgomery Drive to the river and turn right onto West River Drive, which connects with the Benjamin Franklin Parkway.

As you return to your hotel from the Playhouse, you'll see a panorama of city lights, including the illuminated Museum of Art and City Hall. With the sights of twentieth-century Philadelphia fresh in mind, your return to the old city may jolt you into that ambiance that most Philadelphians feel. It's as if there are two cities at times, but at other times one is able to encompass several centuries at once and to feel the breadth of this exciting city—its past, present and future.

## Other Accessible Attractions

Academy of Music, Broad and Locust streets

Academy of Natural Sciences, 19th Street and Benjamin Franklin Parkway

Afro-American Historical and Cultural Museum, 7th and Arch streets

Annenberg Center, 3680 Walnut Street

Christ Church, 2nd and Market streets

Civic Center and Museum, 34th and Spruce streets

Franklin Field, 33rd and Walnut streets

Franklin Institute and Fels Planetarium, 20th Street and Benjamin Franklin Parkway (enter thru parking lot)

Jewish History Museum, 4th and Arch streets

J. F. Kennedy Stadium, Broad Street and Terminal Avenue

Liberty Bell Race Track, Knights Road and Woodhaven Road

Longwood Gardens, Kenneth Square

Mikveh Israel Cemetery

Mummers Museum, 2nd and Walnut streets

National Carl Schurz Foundation

New Hall Marine History Museum

Old St. Mary's Church

Philadelphia Exchange

Presbyterian Historical Society

Robin Hood Dell, East and West, Fairmount Park near 33rd Street

Schuylkill Valley Nature Center, Hagy's Mill Road

Spectrum Stadium, Broad and Pattison streets

St. Peter and Paul Cathedral

Showboat River Tours, Delaware and Race streets
Veteran's Stadium, Broad and Pattison streets
Walnut Street Theater, 825 Walnut Street

INTRODUCING
*Rollin' On* adviser, wheeler Bonnie Gellman

*Title:* Director, Mayor's Office for the Handicapped
*Telephone number:* (215) 686–7120
*Hometown:* Philadelphia
*Favorite tourist site:* Liberty Bell
*Hidden corner:* Tea Garden beside the Second Bank
*Rendezvous:* Kite & Key Room, Benjamin Franklin Hotel
*Offbeat restaurant:* Water Works Cafe
*Place for music:* Grendel's Lair on South Street
*View:* the city as seen from the top of the stairs in front of the
     Museum of Art (accessible from the rear entrance)
*Natural wonder:* Schuylkill River
*Museum:* Philadelphia Museum of Art
*Ramble:* the river walkway at Penn's Landing
*Non-tourist destination:* Italian Market
*Offbeat experience:* Laser show at the Living History Museum
*Traditional restaurant:* Old Original Bookbinder's
*Low-cost restaurant:* one of the 25 food stalls at the Gallery Mall
*Ice cream shop:* Sugar Cone on South 2nd Street
*Reading suggestion: Rebels and Gentlemen* by Carl and Jessica
     Bridenbaugh
*Place to get a wheelchair repaired:* Accurate Medical Services
*Tip on having a great time in Philadelphia:* Take your time, enjoy
     the trees, the people, the sights and sample a blueberry ice
     that you buy from a vendor on the street.

# 9

# San Antonio

Cypress and golden rain trees are your roof, banks of hibiscus and spider lily, your walls. Aboard the river barge, open to the soft night air and scent of magnolia, you cruise on the curving San Antonio River. Along the banks a Dixieland band plays. The colored lights of a dozen outdoor cafes and shops dance on the green river. At a bend the barge turns, leaving the music, laughter, and chatter behind. Before you stretches a bending path of dark water, outlined by the soft, white light that falls from street lamps.

In the quiet night you become a twentieth-century explorer, venturing into unknown worlds. In your mind's eye, vivid pictures of your day's explorations come into view. You see again the yellowed walls of the brooding Alamo, the elegance of old Spain that is preserved in the Spanish Governor's Palace, the fiesta of color and sound that makes up the Mexican Marketplace. You delight again in the fascinating displays and audiovisual shows at the Institute of Texan Culture, the sense of history you discovered in the old La Villita settlement, the beauty of the city parks with their tiled fountains and exotic plantings. You imagine what is yet to come in this most surprising of cities, as the river barge glides to the bank that is the doorway into your riverside hotel. You roll only a few feet when a sidewalk cafe with the lure of a tangy Marguerita bids you stop to sip while watching the parade of boats and people.

Some cities are romantic, others beautiful, historic, friendly, or fascinating. Not many are something of each—and secret, too.

137

What surprises most who visit this Texas city is that its allure is not better known. Has it been kept a secret on purpose by those who want to keep it unspoiled?

You can wonder about this—and also decide if you'll tell anyone about San Antonio yourself—as you explore this city of three-quarters of a million that rambles over 317 square miles. Fortunately for the traveler, sightseeing attractions lie within a five-mile area, with some of the major sites and museums within a few blocks of the tourist hotels.

This compactness, combined with a low-cost public transportation system of wheel-aboard vehicles, means excellent mobility for the wheelchair traveler. In addition, most of the sightseeing attractions are accessible, and a number of hotel and riverside restaurants can also accommodate the wheeler.

Of the several hotels with special wheelchair facilities, the Hilton Palacio del Rio Hotel is situated right on the riverfront, thus enabling the wheeler to board the river barges at his back door. The central location of the hotel also permits self-pushed tours to such nearby attractions as the Arenson River Theater, the old settlement of La Villita, the Transportation Museum, and the Alamo.

But best of all, the San Antonio River and its meandering river walk, the Paseo del Rio, provides the wheeler with unending potential for talking and laughing with the friendly people of San Antonio. For the Paseo del Rio draws not only tourists but the natives themselves, who still live in a world that is relaxed enough to permit the ultimate in nonproductive behavior: strolling for the sake of strolling. San Antonians come to their river in the evening with no purpose but to see it again, to stroll among the tourists and to ride the river barge into the quiet, magnolia-scented night.

## Planning Your Trip

Except for hot August and the cool winter months, you can enjoy San Antonio any time. Best of all is the spring or fall. If you've heard of the famed Fiesta San Antonio, your first thought will be to plan your visit to coincide with this mid-April celebration. Over fifty concerts, shows, exhibitions, pageants, parades and other excuses for merrymaking are staged throughout the city during this ten-day event. Although some of the events, like the Night in Old San Antonio fiesta and the exhibits along the narrow River Walk may be too crowded for most wheelers, others are not. Good bets include the concerts held at the Alamo and the Theater of Performing Arts, the crafts exhibition and demonstrations held at the Southwest Craft Center, the Square and Round Dance Festival staged in the Municipal Auditorium, and the Fiesta Flambeau and Battle of the Flowers parades which can be viewed from various parts of the city.

Another good time for a visit to San Antonio is during June when the accessible Arenson River Theater comes alive with the Sunday night Noche Folklorica and the lively Fiesta Noche del Rio, which is presented on Tuesdays, Fridays, and Saturdays.

October brings the River Art Show, and fall a series of concerts by the San Antonio Symphony at the accessible Theatre for the Performing Arts in the handsome Convention Center.

For information on the city and its attractions, write to the San Antonio Convention and Visitors Bureau, 321 Alamo Plaza, San Antonio, Texas 78205. If history is of interest, you won't want to miss reading the superb historical and pictorial guide *San Antonio* by Charles Ramsdell. It's available from the University of Texas Press, and you can receive a copy by sending $4.95 to them, P.O. Box 7819, University Station, Austin, Texas 78712. In San Antonio you can pick up a copy at Joske's department store or at the Palacio del Rio Hotel.

The first edition of *A Guide to San Antonio for the Handicapped* is available from the Easter Seal Society, 2818 South Pine Street, San Antonio, Texas 78210.

As for packing your bag, rain is possible almost anytime, so pack your rain gear. Also bring your sunshine wearables and a sweater or jacket for cool fall or spring evenings.

To take advantage of the San Antonio Transit System's low-cost Handilift wheelchair conveyance, you'll have to obtain a certificate of eligibility before your arrival. To do this, request that one be issued to you by writing to the San Antonio Transit System, P.O. Box 12489, San Antonio, Texas 78212, or call them at (512) 227–5371. You will receive a form to be filled out and returned. When it is received, the eligibility certificate will be sent to you.

Should time be limited, ask that the certificate be sent to you at the hotel where you'll be staying in San Antonio. Since Handilift runs only on weekdays, plan your trip for weekdays.

## Getting There

San Antonio International Airport, enlarged in 1977, is most accessible from the southeast entrance. Specially designed restroom facilities for wheelchair users are located in the southeast end of the building.

Taxicabs are readily available at the airport. Fares from the airport to the downtown tourist center run about $8. By making advance arrangements, the wheeler arriving at San Antonio airport can use the Handilift for his or her trip downtown (see Planning Your Trip section of this chapter for details).

The San Antonio Railroad Station, 1174 East Commerce Street, is served by Amtrak. Although the station is accessible there are no restrooms especially designed for wheelchair use.

## Getting Around

The Handilift, at 50¢ per ride, can be used instead of taxicabs on weekdays between 6:30 A.M and 6:30 P.M. But first you must obtain your certificate of eligibility (see Planning Your Trip for details), and also you must make your transportation reservation twenty-four hours in advance. Call (512) 922–1234 to make reservations and for additional information.

The Handilifts are the classic lift-equipped vans. Eight vans are currently in the fleet that serves mobilely impaired citizens and visitors. Your request for transportation for the purpose of recreation, of course, will be superceded by requests of greater need. You may find it worth the convenience of using Handilift to make your request by telephone, finding out when you do whether or not you can be accommodated.

Taxicabs in San Antonio are plentiful, with four major operators, including Checker Cab. Rates are $1.45 for the first mile and 60¢ for each additional mile.

The flat terrain of the city, combined with a growing number of curb cuts, makes San Antonio a good destination for the wheeler who likes to ramble on his or her own. Most often, you'll find curb cuts on three out of four corners at an intersection. Alamo Street on the west side is completely curb cut between the HemisFair Plaza and the Alamo. The newly renovated Mexican Market and the stretch of sidewalk that links it with the Spanish Governor's Palace is also well cut. Under a two-year Handicapped Access Program initiated in 1977, the city continues to ramp existing curbs. High priority for ramping are the curbs in Brackenridge Park, particularly those around the San Antonio Zoo.

As for driving yourself, none of the car rental agencies offer cars with hand-controlled devices. If you drive your own car to San Antonio or bring along your own hand controls to be installed on location, you'll find the parking easier than in most cities. Special handicapped parking spaces are offered at most visitor attractions, including the Mexican Market, City Hall across from the Spanish Governor's Palace, within HemisFair Plaza, and at the rear entrance to the Institute of Texan Culture.

## Where to Stay

The **Hilton Palacio del Rio Hotel,** 200 South Alamo Street, may be one of the only hotels in the world with an elevator button marked "River." The hotel's back door opens onto the River Walk and the outdoor El Comedor cafe. All rooms have balconies overlooking the river or city.

Because of its accessibility to the river, the Hilton is top choice for wheelchair travelers. One can roll along the river walk outside the hotel to the next door Durty Nel's pub, and by crossing the river by boat or street-level sidewalk reach the opposite side. On the side opposite the hotel are four accessible restaurants, several nightclubs, and shops.

Other hotels offering rooms especially equipped for the physically disabled include:

Holiday Inn NW, 6023 Northwest Expressway
Holiday Inn NE, 3855 PanAm Highway
Holiday Inn-Downtown, 318 West Durango
TraveLodge NW, 9806 Interstate 10W

Although not offering rooms especially designed for the disabled traveler, two other hotels in San Antonio's sightseeing heart are good accessible possibilities:

The **Menger Hotel,** 204 Alamo Plaza, across the street from the

Alamo was originally built in 1859. The city-block-square hotel offers an ultramodern wing, a lovely patio with swimming pool, and a dining room, and coffee shop.

The **St. Anthony Hotel,** 300 East Travis Street, overlooks Travis Park in the heart of downtown. This gracious old hotel features a grand lobby enhanced by antique furnishings imported from Paris, museum-quality paintings and sculptures, a marble fireplace, and sun-filled Spanish tile veranda. The hostelry's Madrid Room and elegant Charles V restaurants are among the city's finest.

### What You'll See and Do

You'll enjoy the river, its beautiful banks of flowers and trees, its walkway fringe, its barges. When you're not cruising on the river, rambling along its banks, or sipping and munching beside it, you'll discover this varied city. Nearby sightseeing revolves around the Alamo with its museum and garden, the unusual Transportation Museum, the old Mexican quarter with its Farmer's Market and shops, and the Institute of Texan Culture. Short drives from the heart of the city take you to the Lone Star Brewery, famed for its remarkable Hall of Horns, to the charming San Antonio Zoo, and to one or more of the old missions.

To find out what's going on get a copy of *Showboat* and *Scene*, the two free tourist publications available at hotels and restaurants. You can also stop by the office of the San Antonio Visitors' Bureau, across the street from the Alamo, or wave to Alonzo King, the Bureau's official ambassador, who travels the streets in a scooter stocked with maps and informative literature.

For special accessibility questions or problems, call on *Rollin' On* adviser Patsy Alford, who is executive secretary to the director of the Bexar County Easter Seal Society, (512) 699–3911.

When it's lunch or dinner time, you'll have the choice of several riverfront restaurants and the lovely dining rooms at nearby hotels. Among the accessible possibilities:

On the Riverfront

    Casa Rio Mexican Restaurant
    Club Ricardo's

El Comedor, Hilton Hotel
El Quetzal Restaurant, Hilton Hotel
Kangaroo Court
Royal Street Crossing

At the Mexican Market

Mi Tierra Cafe & Bakery
Karam's Kantina

Downtown

Cafe del Sol, La Mansion Motor Hotel, 112 College Street
Charles V Room, St. Anthony Hotel, 300 East Travis Street
Colonial Dining Room, Menger Hotel, 204 Alamo Plaza
G. M. Steak House, 512 East Houston
Joske's Camellia Room and Aztec Patio, 102 Alamo Plaza
Madrid Room, St. Anthony Hotel
Schilo's, 424 East Commerce Street (one step)
Stockman's, 409 East Commerce Street (2 steps)
Tower of the Americas Restaurant, HemisFair Plaza

Elsewhere

Delta Catfish Company, 7075 San Pedro Street (1 step)
Earl Abel's, 4200 Broadway
El Nacho Grande, 1363 Austin Highway
El Rancho Mexican Restaurant, 1326 Goliad Street (1 step)
Gallagher's, 9702 IH 10 West
Hungry Farmer, 2119 Southwest Military Drive
King Wah Restaurant, 1512 Bandera Road
La Louisianne, 2632 Broadway Street (1 step)
Little Red Barn Steak House, 1836 South Hackberry Street
Luby's Cafeteria, 3800 South New Braunfels Street
        4541 Fredericksburg
        252 North Star Mall
Magic Time Machine, 902 Northeast Loop 410 (1 step)
Naples, 3210 Broadway (1 step)
Pan American Mexican Restaurant, 720 Pleasonton Road
Tee Pee Steak House, 1718 Austin Highway (1 step)

## TOUR 1

WHAT YOU'LL DO

- Visit the Alamo, with self-conducted tour, slide presentation.
- Lunch at the Menger Hotel.
* • Visit the Institute of Texan Culture and tour exhibits, see films, demonstrations, and special dome show.
- Dine at Casa Rio and take after-dinner tour along Paseo del Rio.
- Boat cruise.

HOW YOU'LL DO IT

- Push from hotel four blocks to the Alamo.
- Push from Alamo one block to Menger Hotel, 204 Alamo Place.
* • Handilift from Menger Hotel to Institute of Texan Culture, HemisFair Plaza (enter from Bowie Street).
* • Handilift from Institute to Casa Rio, 430 East Commerce Street (enter via Market Street parking lot).
- Boat cruise, then disembark at hotel.

THINGS TO KNOW

- The Alamo open 9:00 A.M–5:30 P.M. Monday–Saturday, 10:00 A.M.–5:30 P.M. Sunday. Free. Long Barracks Museum in northwest corner, mission gardens in rear.
- Menger Hotel serves meals in the Colonial Room, 11:00 A.M–10:00 P.M.
* • Institute of Texan Culture open September–May, 10:00 A.M–4:00 P.M. Tuesday–Friday; 1:00–6:00 P.M. weekends. June–August, Tuesday–Sunday 12:30–6:00 P.M. Admission free. Dome shows: 11:00 A.M., 1:30 and 3:30 P.M.
- Casa Rio open 11:30 A.M.–8:30 P.M. weekdays, Saturday 'til 9:00 P.M.
- Riverboat tours run from 10:00 A.M. to 10:00 P.M., $1. Ask to be let off at Hilton Hotel (one step up to hotel).

* Indicates restriction in time of visit.
† All sites listed under "Restrooms" offer accessible facilities with wide stall doors and grab bars unless otherwise indicated.

* • Handilift must be reserved twenty-four hours ahead, available weekdays only.

RESTROOMS †

• Institute of Texan Culture
• Hilton Hotel

You may feel it appropriate to approach the Alamo slowly and thoughtfully. If you'd like to wheel the four flat blocks from the Hilton Hotel to the Alamo Plaza, you'll see the Cenotaph dedicated to the Alamo defenders some blocks before you arrive.

A good way to understand the **Alamo** with both your head and your heart is to roll first into the Alamo Chapel's Flag Room. Many people believe the town was defended by Texans who were simply protecting their land and their livelihood. Actually, only a few of the two hundred defenders were native Texans or land owners. Most, like David Crockett, owed Texas nothing and had no stake in San Antonio. The flags displayed in the Flag Room represent twenty states and six foreign countries. They tell the tale—that men from throughout the country and the world came to fight tyranny, knowing they would die, but so moved by the spirit of freedom that was sweeping the world that they chose to fight to give others a chance at freedom.

In the book *San Antonio* (see Planning Your Trip for details on ordering a copy), you'll read eyewitness accounts of the battle as told by the young Enrique Esparza and the mother, Susanna Dickinson. The drama, as filled with emotion as any you'll ever read, is evidenced by the objects on display in the chapel. Perhaps you'll hear the strength in Colonel William Travis's voice as you read the words he said when he placed his black stone ring on a string around the neck of Mrs. Dickinson's baby daughter. You'll see the ring and one of the three bells that hung outside the chapel during the battle, and an original Dickert rifle found at the Alamo right after the battle.

Roll inside the sacristy, the small dark room where Mrs. Dickinson and her daughter waited out the thirteen-day siege; some still sense the smoke and roar of battle. You can look, too, for the spot by the door near the north transept where Enrique was hoisted into the Alamo to feel the cold cannon his father tended beneath him.

As you roll through the chapel, you'll see a scale model of the Alamo, paintings representing scenes from the battle, guns and display cases devoted to David Crockett, and more.

Outside the chapel, in a courtyard of stone walls draped in lush vines, stands one of the twelve-pounder cannon used by the Alamo defenders. An ancient oak tree shades the weathered iron emplacement and brushes leaves on the tin roof of the Long Barracks, once the living quarters for priests when the Alamo was only a mission. During San Antonio's world's fair, HemisFair '68, the Long Barracks was renovated to become a museum of Alamo and Republic of Texas history. Here you'll see historic portraits, manuscripts, guns, coins, and a special audiovisual presentation re-creating the Alamo tragedy.

Continuing from the Long Barracks to the rear of the compound, you'll see a remnant of the irrigation canal that once, much wider, served as a moat around the mission. Now the concrete waterway, bright with gold fish, is part of what may be the loveliest garden in San Antonio. Roses and chrysanthemums bloom in season against a backdrop of purple sage, the pale white leaves of locust trees, flowering persimmon, cottonwood, and Japanese yew trees. Notice the unusual huisache, a wispy tree cloaked in delicate yellow flowers.

Forty years after the defeat of the Alamo, when the ruins housed a store and warehouse, "the oasis of Southwest civilization" opened across the street—the **Menger Hotel.**

In 1877 a woman journalist, on seeing the hotel, wrote that she felt as if she were in old Spain. She deemed it "an enchanting spot," summing up that "there is probably nothing like it in America." The fashionable hotel, built on the site of the Menger Brewery, made its own beer and was famous for its wild game dinners and fresh turtle from the San Antonio River.

The original structure has been carefully restored and preserved. You may hear the echoes of jangling spurs and swishing hoop skirts as you roll into the original lobby, and hear a "bully" or two in the bar, where Teddy Roosevelt recruited his cavalry to fight the Spanish in Cuba. The Menger Bar is supposed to be an exact copy of the bar in the British House of Lords.

For lunch visit the **Colonial Dining Room** or the Patio Room, overlooking the hotel's lush tropical garden—complete with alligator pond. You'll want to try Menger's famous golden cheese soup, the poached redfish, and homemade mango ice cream.

Continue from the hotel by Handilift or cab to the **Institute of Texan Culture** on the site of the 1968 San Antonio HemisFair. The fair site is currently undergoing extensive renovation, with various buildings and sites being improved as city funds become available.

The Institute of Texan Culture, not a museum but an educational center, tells the history of Texas through exhibits on the twenty-six different ethnic groups that contributed to its history. It is the first presentation in America of a regional history in which all of the diverse elements of the population are included. Each is given its share of credit for its contribution to the whole. This unique concept gives most visitors an entirely new picture of Texas, and Texans themselves are left with feelings of kinship.

To present the multicultural story dramatically, the Institute uses a variety of techniques. It combines pictorial and three-dimensional elements with light, sound, color, texture, and movement to involve all the senses and create a total environment. For instance, by borrowing relics, paintings, and family treasures, the center created a German section, which has as focus an old-fashioned bandstand draped in bunting. Inside the bandstand are the musical instruments used for making the oompah-oompah music that is heard on the sound system. Important to the presentation is the use of spokespersons in authentic dress who explain the exhibits, tell folk tales related to them, and demonstrate how the artifacts are used.

At the Indian exhibit, interpreter Rocky Stalings, who is part Tonkawa and Cherokee Indian and also part Irish, explains the Indian way of life. At the entrance to his teepee, you sit to hear his explanations of how Indians built their cowhide tepees, made arrowheads and tomahawks, cured buffalo hides, and gambled with painted plum seeds. You touch furry buffalo hides, thump a calfskin tom-tom, and hear the recorded sound of rustling grass, bird songs, and coyote crys.

At the Swedish exhibit you enter a replica of a frontier home to see family treasures and necessities, including a richly illustrated

Bible, a woman's festival dress, rough hand-hewn farm imple-
ments, and a hand-held washing machine.

Other exhibits show the spinning wheel and handmade looms of
the early Norwegians, the festival dragons of the Chinese, a Dutch
wooden windmill, photographs of Negro cowboys, and the armor
of a Spanish conquistador.

All the cultures depicted in the many exhibits are brought together in the Institute's spectacular multimedia presentation. You
sit beneath a huge dome enveloped in sound and the projected
images of thirty-eight movie and slide projectors. On 292 screens
you see the faces and places of Texas, a total panorama of this
state that has been called the bubbling center of the melting pot
that is America.

In order to see it all and enjoy the many experiences that the
Institute offers, be sure to pick up the schedule of daily events.
With careful planning, you'll catch the tepee lecture, a spinning
and tortilla-making demonstration, the multimedia dome show, a
folk music concert, and a general tour of the exhibits.

From the Institute you may want to go directly by Handilift or
cab to San Antonio's famous River Walk, the **Paseo del Rio.** The
side of the river with the most shops and restaurants is accessible
from the parking lot of the **Casa Rio Restaurant.** You'll need assistance rolling down the steep incline that connects the parking lot
with the below-street-level Paseo del Rio. Once at the river side,
however, you'll have a paved, flat walkway leading north for about
two blocks. After passing several restaurants, you'll come to one
narrow portion, a 29-inch passageway between the base of the
Commerce Street Bridge and a building. Beyond it lie several more
restaurants and the interesting **River Square Marketplace.** The first
level of this three-level arcade is accessible. Inside you'll see a
cross section of art and handicraft shops featuring such goods as
rock pictures, hand-crafted leather, metal sculpture, ink drawings,
and silver jewelry.

Among the accessible restaurants along your route is the **Casa
Rio,** with its inexpensive and authentic Mexican cuisine; **Kangaroo
Court,** specializing in fresh seafood; and the **Royal Street Crossing,**
featuring crêpes.

When you're about ready to return to the Hilton Hotel, board

the **river barge** for a cruise of the river. Be sure to tell the captain
that you want to disembark at the Hilton Hotel. As you cruise you
can appreciate the lush plantings that line the river banks. Spider
lilies and hibiscus grow in great profusion under banana, magnolia,
bamboo, golden rain, loquat, and tall ball cypress trees. The lux-
uriant subtropical foliage is replanted in part with the seasons by
the San Antonio Park and Recreation Department, which main-
tains the Paseo del Rio as it would any other city park.

Your river barge first heads south on the horseshoe-shaped river,
passing through the orchestra pit of the **Arenson River Theater.** On
one side of the river you see the grassy rows of theater seats climbing the hillside, and on the other the stage where singers, dancers,
and musicians perform during spring and summer fiestas.

Continuing past the theater, the barge follows the river through
canyons that rise to the buildings of downtown San Antonio. You
pass the Spanish-style **La Mansion Hotel,** the thirty-one-story
Tower Life Building, and the spires of old churches. Then the
barge turns around, retracing its path, finally heading north to the
lagoon that is at the doorway to the modern **Convention Center.**
In 1968 the river was extended to the Center so that delegates
could travel to and from their riverside hotels by water.

As you disembark at the **Hilton Hotel,** you may be lured by the
hotel's inviting sidewalk cafe to sit for a while and enjoy the
sounds of the night. Perhaps with a tangy Marguerita in hand, you
can review your day and anticipate your tomorrow in surprising
San Antonio.

## TOUR 2

WHAT YOU'LL DO

- Visit the Lone Star Brewery, with stops at the Hall of Horns
  and Buckhorn Bar.
- Drive to one or more of the four San Antonio missions.

* Indicates restriction in time of use.
$___/$___ indicates adult/child admission fees.
† All sites listed under "Restrooms" offer accessible facilities with wide
stall doors and grab bars unless otherwise indicated.

- Tour the Mexican Market with its Produce Row, Market Square Building, and Farmers' Market.
- Lunch at Mi Tierra Cafe & Bakery.
- Visit the Spanish Governor's Palace.
- Dine at the El Comedor, with after-dinner libations at Durty Nel's.

### HOW YOU'LL DO IT

* • Handilift or cab to the Lone Star Brewery, Lone Star Boulevard at Roosevelt Street.
- Optional drive to one or more of the four missions.
* • Handilift or cab from the Lone Star Brewery to the Mexican Market, Saba, Santa Rosa, Houston and Commerce streets.
- Push from Mexican Market three blocks to Spanish Governor's Palace, Commerce and Cameron streets.
* • Handilift from Palace to Hilton Hotel.
- Push from hotel next door to Durty Nel's.

### THINGS TO KNOW

- Lone Star Brewery open daily 9:30 A.M.–5:30 P.M. Admission $1/50¢.
- Old Spanish Mission Tour tickets for all four missions $1.
- Mi Tierra Bakery & Cafe open twenty-four hours; no reservations needed.
- Market Square Building open 10:00 A.M.–7:00 P.M. daily.
- Durty Nel's open 11:00 A.M.–midnight daily, 'til 2:00 A.M. Saturday and Sunday.
* • Handilift must be reserved 24 hours ahead, available weekdays only.

### RESTROOMS †

- Mi Tierra Cafe
- Market Square Building, north and south entrances
- Farmers' Market
- City Hall (across from Spanish Governor's Palace)
- Hilton Hotel

The world's record longhorn steer, a 78-point buck whitetail deer, and a 1056-pound black marlin are among the trophies that draw a half million visitors a year to the exhibit halls of the **Lone Star Brewing Company.**

The collection, featuring horned trophies from game animals of the world, was begun in 1884 for the proprietor of San Antonio's famous Buckhorn Saloon and was later moved to the Buckhorn curio shop in downtown San Antonio. The fabulous array of horns and stuffed animals, once buried in the cluttered curio shop, is now fittingly displayed in spacious halls. Artificial and natural lighting, backgrounds of realistic Texan scenes, walls of pine, cypress, and driftwood dramatically showcase the collection for the first time.

You can easily spend hours rolling between the halls devoted to horned animals, birds, fish, firearms, and memorabilia dating back to the early years of the brewery. In the Texas Room, devoted to wildlife specimens native to Texas, note Old Tex, a stuffed deer with a horn spread of more than eight feet. He stands in an autumn scene beneath the room's crowning glory, a chandelier of four thousand horns, weighing three tons. Don't miss such sights as a rare light-colored Asian leopard, quetzal bird, crested pigeon from Australia, Lady Amherst's pheasant of Asia, twenty-five-year-old gorilla, polar and grizzly bears. You'll also want to see the ceiling of deer antlers, the furniture made from horns and skins, pictures made from rattlesnake rattles, and the reproduction of the chalkstone cottage where O. Henry lived during his extended visits to San Antonio. Outside along a breezeway, note the colorful murals of early Texas life and enjoy the extensive grounds that include a German beer garden.

If you're driving or continuing your tour by taxicab, you may want to go two miles south to the first of the four missions lining the Old Mission Trail. The accessible **Mission Concepcion** is the nearest. It is also the best preserved of the Texas missions and the oldest unrestored stone church in the United States. Now a national historic landmark, it is about to be administered by the National Park Service, which means if it doesn't offer park guides to attractions of the site when you are there, it shortly will. The next mission on the Trail is Mission San Jose, operated by the state of Texas and in the process of being made barrier free. The Mission San Francisco de la Espada and San Juan Capistrano are respectively four and six miles farther along the trail. Both are accessible. If you'll be seeing more than one mission, buy the Old Spanish Mission Tour Ticket, which permits you to see all four for $1.

As you approach your next destination, the Mexican Market on the west side of town, you'll pass Main Plaza, center of the city's life since the 1700s. It's been the scene of Indian skirmishes, annunciations of Spanish kings, battles, parleys, crusades, killings, and duels. Nearby Military Plaza, the first permanently settled spot in Texas, once was as lively but definitely more flavorful. Here it was that the "chili queens" set up their stands amidst the fresh vegetables, eggs, poultry, and butter vendors. Today it is marked by City Hall and the Spanish Governor's Palace, which you'll visit after lunch.

With thoughts of chili queens and possibly the scent of wild marjoram and hot chili peppers, lunch may well be on your mind as you reach the **Mexican Market.** This four-block complex of cafes, stores, and shops is one of San Antonio's most recent innovations. A shopping site since the early 1800s, it includes the old Produce Row, the new Market Square Building, and a renovated Farmers' Market. As you ramble along the smooth, flat streets, note the drugstore with a doctor on duty, the food store with mortars, pestles, and washboards in the windows, the unbelievable **Botica de San Pedro** with its love potions, and the lacy white El Mercado building, which was the original Farmers' Market. At **Los Cocos** you can buy such exotic mementoes as canned cactus to mix with eggs; *mole poblano*, a packet of seasonings used for making the famous Mexican chicken dish; and every spice you can think of, including saffron.

In the heart of it all stands the indomitable **Mi Tierra Cafe.** As its name implies, its owners hung onto their restaurant ownership even though all around them shops and restaurants sold out to the city government when the area was recently renovated. Mi Tierra is as individualistic as it is firm. Christmas tree lights twinkle all year round. Tinsel garlands and ornaments celebrate a non-ending festival. At night mariache musicians add to the mood with lively music.

Mi Tierra, open twenty-four hours a day, draws everyone: construction workers in hard hats, businessmen, matrons in sun hats, school kids in jeans, and Mexican-American moms, dads, and youngsters. This is the place to watch people, to hear your favorite Mexican tunes on the individual jukeboxes at each table, and to eat. The menu lists both American and Mexican favorites, including a rich chicken mole, pumpkin bread, and pastry from the cafe's own bakery.

After lunch, wheel across the way to the new **Market Square Building.** Inside you'll find forty-five shops selling every Mexican item you've ever heard of. The shops, decorated with crêpe paper, flags, and banners, contain such treasures as sturdy Yucatan shirts, glazed watermelon and cactus candy, paper flowers, elaborate piñatas, fine antique furniture, colorful pots, onyx chess sets, and ornate leather belts.

Probably you'll have a gay paper flower in your hat and some cactus candy in your pocket when you leave the building and head for the **Farmers' Market** to the west. Here under one huge roof you'll find the choicest of fruits and vegetables in season—fresh Mexican chili peppers, strings of garlic, local pineapples, strawberries, and tomatoes.

If you'd like to wheel the three or four blocks to the Spanish Governor's Palace, do it the easy way with a stop at the delightful **Karam's Kantina** on the edge of Produce Row. Sit in the skylit Greenery, beside stained glass windows, and savor the mood that's reminiscent of Vera Cruz. Sipping a Margarita will amplify the south-of-the-border ambience.

The faithfully restored **Spanish Governor's Palace,** now a national historic landmark, is the only remaining Spanish colonial mansion in Texas. When you enter this home of subdued elegance, you move backward in time into eighteenth-century San Antonio. Candles flicker in the family chapel with its saints painted on wood. You glimpse from the chapel the dining room with its gleaming copper, winecellar cupboard, and vases of dried flowers. In the family bedroom you see a three-hundred-year-old walnut brazier (the room's only source of heat) beside a seventeenth-century carved rosewood bed with twisted posts. The primitive kitchen with its wooden utensils and charcoal brazier opens onto a tiny herb garden.

By leaving the Palace and rolling around the corner on Commerce Street, you can enter the side gate that leads to a delightful patio. Here under old trees you follow stone mosaic paths that are copies of the original ones to an arbor of muscat grapes, a cactus and palm garden, a fountain that tumbles into a pond of water lilies.

You can wait for your cab or Handilift in the city garden that borders the Palace patio. Then, returning to the **Hilton Hotel,** spend some time on the riverfront with dinner at the hotel's outdoor **El Comedor** restaurant and after-dinner drinks at **Durty Nel's,** the hotel's lively indoor-outdoor tavern.

## TOUR 3

WHAT YOU'LL DO

- Visit the Transportation Museum.
- Tour the San Antonio Zoo or the Witte Memorial Museum.
- Lunch and shop on the Paseo del Rio.
- Cruise along the river.
- Explore La Villita.
- Dine at La Mansion Hotel.

HOW YOU'LL DO IT

- Push two blocks from the Hilton Hotel to the San Antonio Museum of Transportation, HemisFair Plaza.
* • Handilift from Museum to San Antonio Zoo, 3903 North St. Mary's Street, or to Witte Memorial Museum, 3801 Broadway Street.
* • Handilift from Zoo or Museum to Casa Rio Restaurant. Enter via parking lot off Market Street.
- Boat cruise to Hilton Hotel.

---

\* Indicates restriction in time of visit.
$___/$___ indicates adult/child admission fees.
† All sites listed under "Restrooms" offer accessible facilities with wide stall doors and grab bars unless otherwise indicated.

- Push from Hilton Hotel two blocks via River Park to La Villita, on Villita Street between Alamo and Presa streets.
- Push a half block from La Villita to Hilton Hotel.
- Cab from Hilton Hotel to La Mansion Hotel, 112 College Street; enter via ramp from garage.
- Cab from La Mansion Hotel to hotel.

### THINGS TO KNOW

* - Handilift must be reserved twenty-four hours ahead, available weekdays only.
- Museum of Transportation open daily 10:00 A.M.–6:00 P.M.
- San Antonio Zoo open daily 9:30 A.M.–6:30 P.M., May–October; 'til 5:00 P.M., November–April. Admission $1/25¢.
- Witte Memorial Museum open weekdays 9:00 A.M.–5:00 P.M.; Sunday 10:00 A.M.–6:00 P.M.
- La Villita shops open Tuesday and Sunday. Colonial Tea Room serves until 3:00 P.M.
- La Mansion Hotel's Cafe del Sol serves dinner from 7:00–10:00 P.M. daily.

### RESTROOMS †

- HemisFair Plaza
- Convention Center
- La Villita

The day begins with visions of galloping horses and dusty trails, as you see Texas' only remaining stagecoach. It continues as you ride through thickets and under statuesque oaks on terrain unchanged since Spanish times. Then you wheel beyond iron gates into a walled village of handcut limestone paths that lead to ancient adobes and flowering courtyards.

The sense that you have journeyed back in time may heighten as you see new portions of this varied city and return again to the now familiar river. By wheeling along the two broad, flat streets that separate the Hilton Hotel and HemisFair Plaza, you'll see at close range the modern Convention Center with its meeting rooms, arena, and theater. Through the broad expanse of windows you'll see the mosaic murals by Juan O'Gorman, the renowned artist who also did the magnificent murals at the University of Mexico.

Just beyond the Center lies the main entrance to HemisFair. Follow the red brick path to the right to the **Museum of Transportation.**

This recently renovated building now displays its fine collection of vehicles in spacious, well-lit rooms. On view are a twenty-passenger mule-drawn trolley car, a vintage 1850 stagecoach that once roughed the remote trails running from San Antonio to Corpus Christi, an 1870 circular hearse, classic and antique automobiles, early bicycles, miniature trains, airplanes, and even a motorcycle.

Concentrating on the rarest of the treasures, admire the only wooden 1903 Roadster in existence, the 1901 DeDion-Boyton that still runs, the 1927 Bugatti racing car, the Pierce Arrow touring car owned by Woodrow Wilson, and a 1930 red Dusenberg convertible coupe valued at $200,000. Before you leave, be sure to see the antique Model T Ford brass head-, side-, and taillamps for sale at the front desk.

Roll to HemisFair Plaza's main entrance on South Alamo Street to rendezvous with that Handilift you ordered yesterday, or go by cab to **Brackenridge Park.** The San Antonio River winds through the 370 acres of oak, magnolia, pecan, and cypress trees. Aside from its few man-made amusements, it remains a woods as idyllic as it was in early Spanish times.

The park offers several accessible attractions: the lily ponds and exotic plantings of the **Oriental Sunken Gardens,** the **San Antonio Zoo,** with its breath-taking exhibit of water fowl and shore birds, and the **Witte Memorial Museum,** one of the major museums in the Southwest. The Zoo is between the other two; the Gardens are three-tenths of a mile to the west; and the Museum one-fourth of a mile to the east. The energetic can, of course, wheel from the destination where the Handilift or cab let them off to one or both of the other sites.

The Zoo boasts a well-rounded collection of birds, mammals, reptiles, and fish scattered in modern habitats over fifty acres of gardens.

Because the Zoo is rather hilly, it's a good idea to plan your routes carefully. Not to be missed is the extensive bird sanctuary to the right as you enter the gate, the equivalent of two long blocks from the entrance. Get someone to assist you up the initial hill, and the remainder of the route will be flat enough. Along the way you'll pass tiny red marmosets, alligators, and Iguana Lizard Island. The water fowl and birds, some caged and some free roaming, live beside beautifully landscaped lagoons and bogs. Note particularly the blue Conre, the hyacinth macaw, and the gray storks.

The **Witte Memorial Museum** offers a diverse exhibit of early American art, American Indian tribal artifacts, natural history habitats, and an important collection of Texas art. The most recent addition is the San Antonio exhibit, with its glittering fiesta costumes and coronation robes. The costumes, which go back to the 1920s, are a fantasy of vibrant silk, lush velvet, and sequins used to draw dazzling pictures of old missions, palm trees, flowers, and dancing señoritas.

A six-screen audiovisual presentation entitled "San Antonio Is . . ." tells of fiesta and the other historic and continuing highpoints of San Antonio life. San Antonians appear in the films to talk about life in this Texas town—both its good and its bad aspects. One speaker seems to sum up the mood of the film presentation when he says simply, "When you leave San Antonio, you're just camping out."

If you've begun your tour early enough, you'll reach the banks of the San Antonio River in time for lunch, perhaps at the **Kangaroo Court.** This indoor-outdoor eatery features inexpensive daily fish dish specials, including shrimp creole, seafood gumbo, and filet Italienne. Note the five different oyster appetizers, the oyster stew, marinated shrimp in a special sauce, and the raspberry cheesecake.

After lunch and browsing at the **River Square,** you'll probably be ready for a daytime cruise along the river, assuming your first one was in the evening. By taking the cruise, you can disembark at the doorway to the Hilton Hotel.

Just around the corner from the hotel lies the old walled La Villita settlement. You can reach it quickly by rolling west to Villita Street and continuing a half block to the right. An alternate route that also gives you a look at a pretty city park is via Market Street to the west of the hotel, then over the Presa Street Bridge to La Villita Street.

If you go the longer route, you'll come to the **Waterboard Park** on the west side of the river. Enter through the gate to see the arbor, fountain, tiled courtyard, and the flowers and cactus.

Continue past the charming stone elephant that marks the entrance to the Hertzberg Circus Collection (inaccessible) to Presa Street, and turn left in the direction of the bridge. Note the "Pajalache Acequia" marker that locates the point where the early water ditch began, continuing south about three miles to Mission Concepcion.

Cross the bridge and you come to the circular **Assembly Hall,** built to blend with the mellowed walls of the Arenson River Theater next to it. Across the street, beyond the lacy gates and limestone walls lies **La Villita.**

Once part of the Alamo mission grounds, the straw-roofed adobe huts served padres and Spanish soldiers. Later, housing German immigrants, the adobe cottages got handsome red tiled roofs and handmade windows, doors, and fancy trim. Revived from decay in the early 1940s, the historic village today houses artists and craftsmen. Within the gaily colored walls of the dozen little houses that make up the village, artists blow glass, weave, throw pots, design jewelry, fashion ceramic tiles, and paint.

Although most of the shops are not accessible, you can look into the **Southwest Craft Center Gallery** and the **Little Studio Art Gallery.** If you have assistance, you can get up the one high step to the porch of the **Colonial Tea Room,** and the friendly church ladies in their calico dresses and bonnets will serve you gingerbread and tea. Beyond one more small step you can enter the tea room with its antiques and tantalizing aromas.

As you roll past the adobe houses, the walls draped in bougainvillea, the tiny side gardens of hollyhocks, and petunias, look for some of the more notable buildings: the two-story Conservation Society Building, built in the 1850s, the Little Church of La Villita, the New Orleans–style Casa Villita cottage, and the pink Cos House where the Mexican general signed articles of defeat in 1835 (which led to Santa Ana's Alamo revenge).

About the same period when the Conservation Society Building and the Cos House were built in La Villita, St. Mary's College moved from its dingy rooms over a livery stable into a new stone building on College Street. You can appreciate the historic college, preserved now as the **La Mansion Motor Hotel.** Take some time to sit in the wood-panelled lobby, which has been preserved to reflect its 1850s appearance. Then dine in the **Capistrano Room**'s glass-enclosed courtyard, choosing from such favorites as Texas T-bone steak, guacamole salad, and mango Bavarian cream. From this vantage you can enjoy the charm of the rare old structure, with its iron balustrades, galleries, and beamed ceilings.

If this is your last evening in San Antonio, the river undoubtedly will call you to its banks. It was the sparkling river that first drew men to this Texas valley. Beside the river oasis they hunted and fished, later building missions, forts and adobes, palaces, and twentieth-century hotels and skyscrapers. Now you, too, are perhaps caught in its spell, not for the life-sustaining food or water it brings, but for its constancy, beauty, and for the world of music and laughter that follows its course on San Antonio's river banks.

## Other Accessible Attractions

Convention Center, HemisFair Plaza
Navarro House, 228 South Laredo Street
Remember the Alamo Theater, Alamo Plaza
San Fernando Cathedral, Main Plaza
Tower of the Americas, HemisFair Plaza

INTRODUCING

*Rollin' On* adviser, wheeler Patsy Alford

*Title:* Executive Secretary, Bexar County Easter Seal Society
*Telephone number:* (512) 699–3911
*Hometown:* San Antonio
*Favorite tourist site:* The Alamo
*Hidden corner:* the patio of the Governor's Palace
*Rendezvous:* Menger Hotel garden
*Offbeat restaurant:* San Francisco Steak House or Magic Time Machine
*Place for music:* Theatre of the Performing Arts
*View:* from atop the Tower of the Americas
*Natural wonder:* the Sunken Gardens in Brackenridge Park

*Museum:* Witte Museum

*Ramble:* Los Patios, a shopping and dining complex set on an old estate

*Non-tourist destination:* San Antonio Symphony pop concerts in Travis Park

*Offbeat experience:* dome show at the Texas Institute

*Traditional restaurant:* Earl Abel's

*Low-cost restaurant:* Luby's Cafeterias

*Ice cream shop:* Baskin-Robbins

*Reading suggestion: A Pictorial & Historical Guide to San Antonio*

*Place to get a wheelchair repaired:* Grayless Mobile Aids Corp. or James' Bicycle Shop

*Tip on having a great time in San Antonio:* Live, eat, drink, people-watch, enjoy nature, shop—spend your time outdoors enjoying the River Walk with its friendly people.

# 10

# San Diego

When you learn that meteorologists voted San Diego the only city in the United States with perfect weather, the other reasons for visiting this vacation city probably seem unimportant. But look at them anyway: this oldest of California cities boasts the world's largest zoo, largest outdoor organ, largest tuna fleet, and one of the world's three greatest hotels. It also claims the country's first mission and her largest mission, oldest iron sailing vessel, and one of America's most visited national monuments. As if that's not enough, San Diego boasts the country's first regularly scheduled city bus with wheelchair lifts.

Does it matter that the city also has one of the world's most beautiful natural harbors, seventy miles of beaches, a 4600-acre aquatic park, an Old Town that's a state historic park, the prototype of all future space theaters, and a hotel that's a historic landmark?

Even without the superlatives, San Diego has lots to offer. Although it's America's ninth-largest city, its air is clear, streets are clean, its people are hometown friendly. Wherever you look there seems to be a view of water: the Pacific Ocean; the crescent-shaped harbor; or Mission Bay Park, the man-made playland of islands and waterways.

Cabrillo National Monument, on the bluffs of Point Loma, overlooking the site where the Spanish explorer stepped ashore proclaiming his discovery of California, affords an unsurpassed vista.

Perhaps its dramatic situation accounts for the monument receiving more visitors than the Statue of Liberty!

Balboa Park, with its Spanish Renaissance buildings from the Panama-Pacific Exposition, offers a wealth of museums, theaters, exhibit halls, and natural beauty. Its neighbor, the San Diego Zoo, attracts three-and-a-half million visitors a year, followed closely by Sea World, a popular marine life entertainment park.

To the north of San Diego stretches the wildly beautiful La Jolla shoreline and artists' community. Across its curving bay bridge lies Coronado, with its Victorian masterpiece, the Hotel del Coronado.

Culture lives in San Diego, too. The city is proud of its new San Diego Convention and Performing Arts Center, home for local opera, symphony, and two ballet companies. The San Diego Civic Light Opera Company presents a series of "starlight opera" productions in the Balboa Park Bowl, while the Old Globe Theatre in Balboa Park is the site for a yearly National Shakespeare Festival.

The wheelchair traveler visiting San Diego gets a sneak preview of what the future holds as far as accessible mass transportation is concerned. In 1977 the city became the first to fit its buses with wheelchair lifts. The five buses now in this new regular service provide service for 75 percent of the population, linking the homes of 900,000 passengers with eighteen shopping centers, ten employment centers, nineteen hospitals, and nine colleges and universities.

The city's Dial-a-Ride service provides another option for the wheelchair sightseer. This fleet of lift-equipped vans can be used for trips from downtown San Diego to the zoo, Old Town, and other attractions.

Good transportation, an abundance of cultural offerings, plus parks and seacoast vistas are all there for the wheeler to discover. Perhaps no other city is as near to being barrier free, to being really yours.

### Planning Your Trip

Although days in San Diego are generally mild and sunny, the December-to-March period is when the area gets most of its 9.11

inches of annual rainfall. But winter still is better in San Diego than most other places, and also in winter you may see a migrating whale. Summer is most popular, with constant sunshine and low humidity. As in other vacation cities, however, summer is the most crowded time of the year in San Diego, but still not congested, because there's plenty of room. You can enjoy the city comfortably in summer with lots of good company, and have it more to yourself in the fall or spring. When it gets down to it, anytime's a good time to visit San Diego.

If you choose summer, you'll be in town for the annual National Shakespeare Festival, which runs from June through mid-September. Three Shakespearean plays in repertory are presented in the Old Globe Theatre,* a recreation of the original Shakespeare theater in England. Renaissance music, dance, and revelry precede each performance on the greensward in front of the theater.

Fall brings the September Piano Festival, when a thousand youngsters play on 101 pianos in a mass recital; the October San Diego Opera season; and the San Diego Symphony season, which runs from October through May.

Other outstanding events around which you can plan your visit include the Pacific Coast Soaring Championships in March, the Old Town Art Fiesta in June, and the Navy Air Show and Open House in October that features demonstrations by the Blue Angels.

As for packing your bag, include sun lotion, sunglasses and a straw hat. Since San Diego is a casual resort city, you needn't bring your finery. Do bring a warm jacket or sweater, however, for the cool evenings.

Write ahead to the San Diego Convention and Visitors Bureau for their fine packet of tourist materials. Address your request to them at 1200 Third Avenue, Suite 824, San Diego, California 92101. The Mission Bay Information Center also sends out information and maps. You can receive their selection by sending your request to them at 2688 East Mission Bay Drive, San Diego, California 92109.

*A Step in Time: San Diego Guide for the Handicapped* is available for 30¢. Send your request to the Junior League of San Diego, 1549 El Prado, Balboa Park, San Diego, California 92101.

* burned in 1978

## Getting There

San Diego International Airport, served by the major airlines, is a one-level modern facility. Although restrooms are accessible and one stall has a 25-inch wide door, none of the stalls are specifically designed for wheelchair use. The airport is located in the center of town, with Harbor Island hotels only minutes away; the downtown hotels are but a five-minute cab ride away.

San Diego is also served by Amtrak. However, because of the low loading platform at the Santa Fe Railroad Station, boarding or disembarking from the trains in a wheelchair is not recommended.

The San Diego Greyhound terminal at First and Broadway Street in the heart of downtown is accessible, but it has no accessible restrooms.

## Getting Around

Except for La Jolla and Coronado, most of the San Diego the tourist wants to see is located within a compact area. This means you'll probably come out ahead using taxicabs, Dial-a-Ride, and the wheelchair-accessible city buses. The one exception will be the day you rent a car to drive to La Jolla and Coronado.

Both Avis and National rent hand-controlled cars in San Diego (see Chapter 2 for details on making reservations). Also, a city-operated Dial-A-Ride service for the handicapped is available to tourists. The twenty-one-bus fleet—each bus can accommodate two wheelchairs—travels within a prescribed zone. The zone does not include the popular resort areas such as Harbor Island, Shelter Island, Mission Bay Park, or La Jolla. The bus does transport by priority those who make reservations from and to such locations as the airport, Mission San Diego de Alcala, the San Diego Zoo, and Old Town. Dial-a-Ride operates from 9:00 A.M. to 5:00 P.M., but you can make reservations anytime between 8:00 A.M. and 6:00 P.M. by calling (714) 232–6871. Fare is 25¢ per one way trip.

Should you stay in downtown San Diego, you may also find it practical to sample the city's regularly scheduled bus service that allows wheelers to ride the bus without getting out of their chairs.

Two routes, both with stops downtown, are available. One goes to the zoo and the other through the lovely Mission Hill area of the city. For schedules and information call 239–8161.

Because the portions of the city you'll be visiting are almost entirely flat, getting around on your own should be a breeze. San Diego is currently in the process of having ramps built into all of its sidewalks. Three hundred and seventy-five new ones were added in 1977, and 270 more are projected for completion by March 1978. Presently most of the downtown area is completed—and a good deal of La Jolla. The waterfront Embarcadero remains uncut in part, so when rolling in that area you'll need assistance.

## Where to Stay

A great many of San Diego's hotels can accommodate wheelchairs, although they are not specifically designed for the disabled. This means you can, with a letter or phone call, let the manager know what your needs are, and often arrangements can be made to fill them. So, if you've heard of a hotel where you'd like to stay, give it a try, and most likely something can be worked out.

Of those hotels that offer specifically designed wheelchair facilities, three are on Harbor Island, and one is on Mission Bay.

The **Sheraton Hotel–Airport** at 1380 Harbor Island Drive and the **Sheraton Hotel–Harbor Island** at 1590 Harbor Island Drive both offer the usual Sheraton amenities. Both are on the water, with lovely grounds and public rooms. If you're the kind who enjoys a ramble beside the water at sunset, however, the Sheraton–Harbor Island offers access to the lovely Spanish Landing Park walkway. You can roll for a mile or more on the flat, wide path, enjoying the boats, the view of the city, and the park itself.

Both the Sheraton Hotel–Airport and the **TraveLodge Tower at Harbor Island,** 1960 Harbor Island Drive, are across a busy street from the Spanish Landing walkway, thus inaccessible because of traffic. However, the view from either is lovely. Both offer rooms with views, rooftop lounges with panoramic views, swimming pools, and restaurants. Each room at the TraveLodge has its own balcony.

The **San Diego Hilton** at 1775 East Mission Bay Drive is a resort with its own private beach, boat dock, Olympic-sized swimming pool, extensive grounds, and public rooms.

Although not specifically designed for wheelchair visitors, these other San Diego hotels can accommodate disabled guests:

> Howard Johnson's, 4544 Waring Road
> TraveLodge, 1201 West Hotel Circle
> TraveLodge, 1305 Pacific Highway
> Bahia Motor Hotel, 998 Mission Bay Drive
> Shelter Island Inn, 2051 Shelter Island Drive
> Royal Inn, 4875 Harbor Drive
> Royal Inn of La Jolla, 7830 Fay Avenue
> Town & Country Hotel, 500 Hotel Circle
> El Cortez Hotel, Seventh and Ash streets
> Islandia Hotel, 1441 Quivira Road

## What You'll See and Do

You'll view the water. Actually you'll do lots more, but the water will never be long out of sight. An important part of your visit will be enjoying it from a waterside walkway, from a bayside restaurant, and from panoramic vistas. Although your days will be filled with beautiful art, fascinating museums, zoos, and parks, your evenings can revolve around the twinkle of city lights reflected on the bay. To enjoy it while dining or sipping, choose from the accessible restaurants listed here, all with watery views:

> Anthony's Fish Grotto, Ash and Harbor Drive
> Atlantis, 2595 Ingraham Street (use side entrance)
> Elario's, Summer House Inn, 7955 La Jolla Shores Drive
> Harbor Seafood Market, Market Street at Harbor Drive
> Mr. A's, 2550 Fifth Avenue
> Red Sails Inn, 2614 Shelter Island Drive
> Reuben E. Lee, 880 Harbor Island Road (ground-floor restaurant only)
> Sky Room, El Cortez Hotel, Seventh and Ash streets
> Tarintio's, 5150 Harbor Drive
> Top of the Cove, 1216 Prospect Street

Other accessible restaurants include:

> Anthony's Fish Grotto, 886 Prospect Street, La Jolla
> Boom Trenchard's Flare Path, 2888 Pacific Coast Highway
> Botsford's Old Place, 1225 Prospect Street, La Jolla (take the elevator to the second floor)
> Caesar's, 5010 Mission Center Road; 5403 Grossmont Center Drive, La Mesa
> Cafe del Rey Moro, 1549 El Prado, Balboa Park
> Chinaland, 3135 Midway Drive (wheelchair-designed restroom)
> Casa Pedrorena, 2616 San Diego Avenue (enter from Congress Street)
> La Valencia Hotel patio, 1132 Prospect Street, La Jolla
> Hamburguesa, 4016 Wallace Street (Old Town)
> Schnitzelbank, 1037 Prospect Street, La Jolla
> Su Casa, 6738 La Jolla Boulevard

Good sources of information for what's going on in town are the free *Reader*, available at newsstands; *Where* and *Today in San Diego*, which you can pick up in hotel lobbies; and the Convention Bureau's quarterly *What's Doing* brochure.

For special wheeler information, call *Rollin' On* advisers Marene and Red Aulger at (714) 582–7648. Marene teaches independent-living classes for the handicapped, and Red is the leading force behind the local Indoor Sports Club chapters.

## TOUR 1

WHAT YOU'LL DO

- Cruise around San Diego Bay.
- Lunch on the waterfront.
- Tour San Diego Zoo.
- See the show at the Reuben H. Fleet Space Theater and Science Center.
- Dine with a view at the El Cortez Hotel.

---

\* Indicates restriction in time of visit.

\$___/\$___ indicates adult/child admission fees.

† All sites listed under "Restrooms" offer accessible facilities with wide stall doors and grab bars unless otherwise indicated.

HOW YOU'LL DO IT

- Cab from your hotel to Harbor Excursion, Broadway at Harbor Drive.
- Wheel two flat blocks from Harbor Excursion to Anthony's Fish Grotto, Harbor Drive at Ash Street; or wheel about a quarter mile to the Harbor Fish Market, Market Street at Harbor Island Drive.
- * • Go by Dial-a-Ride from Anthony's to the San Diego Zoo, Balboa Park, or board the #7 lift bus at Market and California Street.
- Push from the zoo to Space Theater and Science Center, El Prado, Balboa Park (use rear entrance).
- Cab from Theater to El Cortez Hotel, Seventh and Ash streets.
- Cab from El Cortez Hotel to your hotel.

THINGS TO KNOW

- Two-hour cruises depart at 10:00 A.M and 2:00 P.M. Cost: $4:50/$2.25.
- Anthony's serves lunch from 11:30 A.M.; open 'til 8:30 P.M.
- Harbor Seafood Mart restaurants open for lunch.
- Lift-service city bus leaves corner of California and Market Street at 1:10 or 2:00 P.M.
- * • Dial-a-Ride must be reserved twenty-four hours ahead and is available only on weekdays.
- Zoo open 8:30 A.M.–6:00 P.M. July–Labor Day; 9:00 A.M.–5:00 P.M. Labor Day–November and May–June; 9:00 A.M.–4:00 P.M. November–May. Admission $3/$1.
- Space Theater shows 11:30 A.M., hourly from 1:00–5:00 P.M. and at 7:30 and 8:30 P.M. Show lasts 50 minutes. Admission $2.75/$1.50, which includes admission to Science Center.
- El Cortez Sky Room serves dinner 5:30 P.M.–12:30 A.M. Reservations advised.

RESTROOMS †

- San Diego Zoo, under Golden Eagle restaurant
- Space Theater and Science Center

Down to the sea in ships and off to outer space in a theater, with time out for a visit with a thousand furry, feathery, and scaley friends. Sightseeing is most fun when there's variety. This is a day filled with sea breezes to refresh the mind, antics of animals to tickle the fancy, and a simulated space voyage to expand consciousness. You'll sample some of each aboard a Harbor Excursion tour boat that circles San Diego Bay, then visiting the world-famous San Diego Zoo, and then by attending a show at the revolutionary Reuben H. Fleet Space Theater.

First stop is the Broadway pier at the foot of Broadway Street at the Embarcadero. Roll out on the pier a few feet for an eye-opening survey of the busy bay, then proceed to the dock, where **Harbor Excursion** tour boats are welcoming passengers aboard.

Lines are cast off, and with a toot of the ship's whistle the excursion boat joins the orderly procession of fishing boats, sailboats, yachts, and merchant ships on San Diego Bay. Sitting inside a glass-enclosed cabin, you hear your guide telling you about this beautiful natural harbor.

The 22-square-mile San Diego Harbor is home port for the world's largest tuna boat fleet and is headquarters for the largest naval fleet in the continental United States. Amidst the submarines, destroyers, giant aircraft carriers, and support ships glide a flurry of white sailboats, an occasional rowboat, and a steady stream of sportsfishing and other motorized pleasure craft.

You can wave at the sailors and sportsmen as you follow a twenty-five-mile route around the crescent bay. During the two-hour cruise you'll pass along the palm-lined Embarcadero waterfront, with its string of tuna seiners, their nets festooned with floats hanging from masts and booms. Alongside them reign three *grande dames* of the sea: the century-old *Star of India* windjammer; the first propeller-driven ferryboat on the West Coast, the *Berkeley*; and the luxury yacht *Medea*, with its gleaming teak exterior.

Passing man-made Shelter and Harbor islands, your excursion boat continues to Ballast Point, the site where Juan Rodriguez Cabrillo first landed on the west coast of the United States in 1542. Above are the green slopes of Point Loma, with Cabrillo National Monument on its southwest tip.

As the cruiser turns around at the borders of the Pacific Ocean, you pass Zuniga Jetty, abounding with sea life. Here pelicans, sea gulls, and cormorants swoop and dive on fishing expeditions. Occasionally one spots a seal lying on a mooring buoy.

Along the shore of North Island you see the Naval Air Station with its giant aircraft carriers come into view. Then your boat goes under the graceful curve of the San Diego–Coronado Bay Bridge for a look at the 32nd Street Naval Station, the Hotel del Coronado, and the broad beaches of the Silver Strand. Heading back to the dock, the boat passes the modern tuna canneries and the old-fashioned Harbor Fish Market.

Once on shore again, you can ramble along the waterfront, either going south about one-fourth of a mile to the Harbor Fish Market or two blocks north to Anthony's Fish Grotto.

The **Harbor Fish Market,** a new seafood processing and dining facility, includes a restaurant, two fast-service seafood bars, live and processed seafood displays, retail sales outlets, coffee and gift shops. For lunch here you might try San Diego's famous abalone or another seafood favorite and enjoy your meal outside, overlooking the bay.

As a luncheon alternate, wheel along the Embarcadero to **Anthony's Fish Grotto,** a four-star restaurant, according to the *Mobil Guide.* Mrs. Ghio, the eighty-five-year-old owner of the famous seafood house, still keeps an eye on food preparations and continues to refuse anyone the secret of her famous fish batter.

After lunch, go by Dial-a-Ride from Anthony's to the Zoo, or if you're lunching at the Harbor Fish Market, roll across the street to California and Market streets to board the #7 lift-service bus that comes by at 1:10 and 2:00 P.M. (check times by calling 239–8161). The bus will take you close to the entrance to the world-famed **San Diego Zoo** in Balboa Park.

Once inside you may wonder if you're in a zoo with lots of flowers and trees, or in a garden with lots of birds and animals. For as you ramble over some of the 123 acres of grounds, you'll see a remarkable array of botanical species. The blossoms of the South African aloes brighten the habitat of the gazelle and elephant. Fifty-foot red flowering trees from Madagascar line the path of Cascade Canyon, where Madagascar red frogs live. A valuable collection of cycads decorates the entrance to the hummingbird aviary. Golden trumpet trees add color to the Reptile Mesa. Orchid trees covered with white blossoms flower beside the hippo pools. Over 2500 species of plants cover the Zoo grounds, which are divided into temperate, tropical, and subtropical transitional zones and into sections where palms and conifers grow.

Some of the plants provide part of the diet of the 4,000 animals living in this flower garden. Begun in 1916 with a small group of animals left after the Panama-Pacific Exposition, the San Diego Zoo now boasts the world's largest collection of wild animals. Some of the 1,100 animal species can be seen nowhere else in captivity: the cuddly koalas from Australia, the long-billed kiwis from New Zealand, the wild Przewalski's horses from Mongolia, and the diminutive pigmy chimps from central Africa. The Zoo also offers the largest collection of parrots in the world, and has an outstanding primate and Australian fauna collection. Hundreds more cages, barless enclosures, houses, aviaries, and ponds are homes for such ever-popular favorites as monkeys, lions, tigers, bears, elephants, and giraffes.

Set within a terrain of mesas and canyons, the Zoo is both hilly and level. You can with planning concentrate on the level areas, or with assistance go downhill and use the two speedramps that carry people uphill. These moving sidewalks measure 27 inches at their base, with side enclosures that fan out at an angle, thus providing more space at the handrail level. If your chair's wheel tracks don't exceed 27 inches, you can be pushed aboard and have enough room for your arms to rest on the chair arms. The two speedramps, which face one another, are near the tiger habitat.

The best route, if you want to stick to level terrain, is the one circling the elephant and giraffe habitats, the bird-monkey-ape complex behind the flamingo lagoon, and the stretch between the Children's Zoo, the Wegeforth Bowl, and the alligator enclosure. Between these three level areas stretches the Zoo's main entrance route, with its shops, the Golden Eagle Restaurant (with its outdoor terrace), the penguin and koala exhibits.

When it's time for a rest, head for the Wegeforth Bowl to see the sea lion show (check for times when you enter). Next to the Bowl lies the delightful Children's Zoo, built to the scale of four-year-olds. Here children pet sheep, pigs, and donkeys, ride huge turtles, rub noses with baby antelope, watch hatching baby chicks, and see newborn animals cared for in the glass-fronted Zoo nursery.

If you have assistance or a good supply of energy, you may want to wheel from the Zoo to the Reuben H. Fleet Space Theater and Science Center, which is the equivalent of two blocks away. By exiting near the Children's Zoo and crossing the parking lot, you'll reach a walkway that borders the Spanish Village. The courtyard of this village of artists' studios is rough and sloping, so you may want just to look from the arched entranceway.

Beyond the village lie formal English gardens under a spreading fig tree, and next to the gardens is the Natural History Museum. Opposite its front entrance on the main park thoroughfare, El Prado, is the **Reuben H. Fleet Space Theater and Science Center.**

If you leave the Zoo by 4:30 P.M. you'll be able to make the 5:00 P.M. show at the Center. Buy your ticket first thing and then spend your time in the Science Center.

The Space Theater has been called a new entertainment medium, the first theater-planetarium, the vehicle by which we *all* can explore outer space. The experience it provides is dazzling, unique, indescribable. You actually sit inside the hemisphere projection screen, surrounded by color, light, sound, and images. Via 70-millimeter Ominmax motion pictures, a sound system with ninety-six speakers, slide projectors, lasers, and a starfield projector, you are taken along as Mariner, Viking, and Pioneer space ships set out on their journey through the stars. Star of this spectacle is the computer-controlled starfield projector, which can create on the screen the stars, moons, and planets as they would appear from any given point in space at any period of time.

The Science Center adjoins the theater and features exhibits on sensory exploration and perception, aimed at providing insight into science through personal involvement in controlled experiments. A heartbeat oscilloscope, a cloud chamber, sand pendulums, image tracers, light-mixing booth, revolving trapezoid, hologram, and laser are among the exhibits that the visitor can operate.

What could possibly follow a trip out to the stars at San Diego's new Space Theater? Why a soaring trip by glass-enclosed elevator to the Sky Room of the hilltop **El Cortez Hotel** in downtown San

Diego. Since the hotel is near Balboa Park and probably en route to your hotel, this is a good time to enjoy one of the best of the city's viewing points, where you can also sip. Enjoy a leisurely drink, hopefully holding out through twilight, then continue your evening with dinner at one of the accessible restaurants listed in the first part of this chapter.

## TOUR 2

WHAT YOU'LL DO

* • Visit the La Jolla shops, galleries, and Museum of Contemporary Art (closed Mondays), with lunch at La Valencia Hotel patio restaurant.
• View the ocean and cliffs along La Jolla Shores and ramble in the oceanside park.
• Explore Mission Bay, with its hotels, marinas, parks, and waterway.
• Visit Cabrillo National Monument, with golf-cart trip to the lighthouse.
• Sightseeing tour of Shelter Island and twilight ramble along the water's edge.
• Dinner at the Del Coronado Hotel.

HOW YOU'LL DO IT

• Drive from hotel to downtown La Jolla, then along the Coast Boulevard, with a stop at Scripps Park.
• Drive from La Jolla through Mission Bay, then along the Ocean Beach Freeway to Sunset Cliffs Boulevard to the Cabrillo Monument.
• Drive from Cabrillo to Shelter Island.
• Push along Shelter Island bay walkway.
• Drive from Shelter Island to Coronado Island and the Del Coronado Hotel, 1500 Orange Avenue.
• Drive from the Del Coronado Hotel to your hotel.

* Indicates restriction in time of visit.
† All sites listed under "Restrooms" offer accessible facilities with wide stall doors and grab bars unless otherwise indicated.

THINGS TO KNOW

* • La Jolla Museum of Contemporary Art open Tuesday–Friday 11:00 A.M.–5:00 P.M., weekends 12:30–5:00 P.M., Wednesday eve 7:00–10:00 P.M. Closed Monday. Donations.
• La Valencia Hotel patio open 7:30 A.M. to midnight. Reservations not necessary.
• Cabrillo Monument open 9:00 A.M.–5:15 P.M., except during the summer, when hours are extended to 7:45 P.M.
• Del Coronado Hotel's Coronet Room serves all day. No reservations required.

RESTROOMS †

• La Jolla Trust & Savings Building, 1225 Prospect Street
• Mission Bay Park, New Bonita Cove near Ventura Bridge
• Cabrillo National Monument

The ocean churns. Foamy crests rise. Waves crash on dark, jagged rocks. Salt spray dances to rest on sandstone palisades. In quiet coves, sapphire water as clear as glass laps curves of warm sand. Weathered beach cottages with colored roofs climb up hillsides carpeted in bougainvillea and oleander, shaded by cedars and pines.

Artists will tell you that the vista of land and sea along the La Jolla coast is the most beautiful, dramatic, and changeable on earth. They prove their point with the paintings you see in dozens of La Jolla's galleries. Scenes of the sea, rocks, cliffs, and lush hillsides come in the shades of gray fog, sunlit days, or the pale glow of sunset. Other paintings show the ocean as a ferocious force carving caves from rock and pounding cliffs to sand. Alongside, the same wild ocean calms to tickle the toes of laughing babies or to touch softly waterside flowers. Whether you're an artist or not, bring with you on this visit to La Jolla an artist's eye for color, contrasting textures and evasive moods.

For a quick trip from your hotel to La Jolla, first get yourself on Interstate 5, the San Diego Freeway, heading north. Take the Ardth Road exit, which sweeps down the mesa to become Torrey Pines Road. The famed **Scripps Institution of Oceanography,** with its **Vaughn Aquarium,** is to the right on La Jolla Shores Drive. The aquarium makes a worthwhile stop, with its interesting tidal pool exhibit, the underwater displays of the La Jolla kelp beds and Mission Bay sea life. The "Under Sea TV" shows what life is really like two hundred feet below the surface of the water.

Follow Torrey Pines Road a few blocks to Prospect Street, which curls into downtown La Jolla. Then get onto Coast Boulevard for a look at the coast artists rave about. Your route will follow Coast Walk, a paved, level walkway that skirts the sea. You may want to choose a favorite portion and roll along it in your chair to enjoy the sea air and vistas better.

As you drive along, you'll see **La Jolla Cove,** one of the most popular spots for skin diving because of its exceptionally clear water. Beyond the piece of land called Alligator Head, which juts into the water, lies Boomer Beach, a surfboarding area. The spacious **Ellen Browning Scripps Park** is a delight, with its wispy palms, acres of grassy parkland, and borders of yellow-flowering sea fig. More and different views open up as you continue south along Coast Boulevard past Shell Beach, Seal Rock, and Whale View Point.

Coast Boulevard turns into Prospect Street near Whispering Sands Beach. Turn left and head north, back in the direction you've just come from for a look at the mission-style **La Jolla Museum of Contemporary Art.** The buildings across the street were designed by the same architect, Irving Gill, who earned a national reputation for his early twentieth-century modern style. Enter via the courtyard, with its fragrant sycamore trees, to see the avant-garde twentieth-century artwork it displays. Don't miss the Museum book shop, its large windows overlooking the sea.

From the Museum drive about four blocks to the heart of town, Prospect and Girard Avenue. You can roll up one side of Prospect, heading north, and return on the other side, heading south. If you do, you'll see a fascinating variety of shops, galleries, and restaurants, many of which are accessible.

Before you begin you may want to stop for lunch at the charming **La Valencia Hotel**'s Spanish-style outdoor cafe. Enjoy a sandwich or salad beneath the pink umbrellas beside a tiled fountain bordered by flowers and ferns.

After lunch, roll into the hotel lobby to see the lovely Spanish tile-topped tables, wrought iron chandeliers, iron gates and screens, the Persian rugs, and huge flower arrangements.

As you explore the courtyards, gardens, and shops on **Prospect**

**Street,** don't miss a look into the **Top of the Cove** restaurant, a re-modelled nineteenth-century La Jolla cottage. At the **London Asso-ciates** shell shop across the street, look for the unusual angel-wing calcite, the fossils, and giant clam shells. The sand castings of sand dollars and fossils on the walls were made in La Jolla.

Almost next door is the colorful **Schnitzelbank,** a German res-taurant serving sausages, sauerkraut, homemade noodles, German home fries, light and dark Riterbrau beer on tap, and more. The **Tarbox Gallery,** a few doors away, shows a broad spectrum of arts by locals—everything from sculptures and paintings, to enamels, pottery, and wood inlay.

Dozens more food, clothing, gift, and garden shops line Girard Avenue. The Spanish-style Arcade Building will lead you back to Prospect Street via the Cove Realty, where you can choose a new La Jolla home from the photos in the windows. Around the corner on Prospect Street, look into the windows of the **Indian Arts and Crafts** shop.

After you've savored La Jolla, continue your tour with a drive along La Jolla Boulevard to Mission Boulevard and Mission Bay Park.

**Mission Bay Park** is a man-made wonder. Twenty years of dredg-ing and developing, at the cost of nearly $60 million, have turned this former marsh into one of the world's great water resorts. Con-tained in the 4600-acre playground are coves, bays, channels, is-lands, nineteen beaches, and twenty-seven miles of shoreline. Mod-ern hotels with windows and cafes overlooking the bay add to its enjoyment, as do the many palm-lined walkways that open up por-tions of its banks to wheelchair travelers. By driving along West Mission Bay Drive and Ingraham Street, you'll see some of its finest points, but for a real in-depth view, plan on stopping for a ramble or at least a long view from the car. Among the possibilities is the spectacular view from the Mission Bay Visitor Information Center, Claremont and East Mission Bay Drive.

Most delightful of all the bay-touring options, however, is a stop at the waterside **Barefoot Bar** at the **Vacation Village Hotel.** You roll to an open-air bar along a wood plank walkway lined with sandalwood trees and petunias. As you sip, your view is of the sparkling blue bay, its fringe of green palm trees, the graceful boats gliding into port or setting off for distant ports like the Bahia Hotel, a mile or two away.

Breathtaking views of the Pacific Ocean are part of any visit to the **Cabrillo National Monument,** which can be the next stop on your tour. The Cabrillo National Monument is the most visited national monument in the country. You'll understand why when you experience its easy accessibility and unsurpassed beauty. To reach it follow Sunset Cliffs Drive to Nimitz Boulevard, then to Chatsworth and onto Catalina (Route 209). From the glass-enclosed Visitors' Center or patio behind, you'll survey the Pacific Ocean, San Diego Harbor, and the city. Below you is Ballast Point, where Rodriguez Cabrillo in 1542, having sailed into the almost hidden mouth of a great bay, tied up his tiny Spanish vessel. The monument commemorates his discovery of California. In several buildings you'll get a push-button history of the bay, see exhibits about Cabrillo and other Spanish explorers, and be able to pick out various warships and planes around the harbor by using identification plaques. Outside reigns a handsome statue of Cabrillo sculpted in sandstone. Behind the statue is the best view of all.

If you'd like to visit the Old Point Loma Lighthouse, which has been restored to look the way it did in 1887, there are electric golf carts available to convey you up to the hilltop site. Just before you reach the lighthouse, you'll come to a plaza where you can see engraved pictures and listen to a recording telling of its history.

While viewing the bay from the Monument you may notice **Shelter Island,** linked to the city by a narrow causeway. The island rose from the sea in the 1940s, when the city began dredging the bay and dumping the surplus on a shoal. Later it added more dredgings to the former mud bank and, *voilà*, Shelter Island. Today the island is an elegant salty paradise of yacht dealers, ship chandleries, sailmakers, marinas, shipyards, hotels, restaurants, parks, and lovely bayside walks. Drive around it to see the Bell of Friendship at the tip, the Polynesian garden and its fountains, bridges, bamboo, and waterfalls, the fishing pier, and the modern hotels. Stop, if time permits, for a ramble along the shoreline walkway, and cap it off with a drink in one of the outdoor restaurants, perhaps the **Bali Hai Restaurant.**

For dinner you can choose to overlook the water from the popular **Tarantino Restaurant** on North Harbor Drive, sampling their famous home fries and generally enjoying a fine meal at a moderate price. Or you can venture across the bay to one of the National Historic Landmarks, the **Hotel del Coronado,** an exceptional example of Victorian grandeur.

To reach the hotel, follow Harbor Drive to Grape Street, get onto Interstate 5 and follow it to the Coronado Bridge exit. Cross the bridge and follow State Highway 75 to the hotel.

Since its opening in 1887 the Hotel del Coronado has been the luxury resort of kings, presidents, and show business personalities. It has played host to eight presidents and was the site of the grand ball where the Prince of Wales reputedly met the woman for whom he later gave up his crown. The main wooden building, surounding a one-and-a-half-acre central courtyard, presents an unforgettable silhouette of towers, parapets, covered walkways, and hand-hewn wooden columns.

Inside you'll see a beautiful gilded cast-iron elevator and the Crown Room's high arched ceilings of natural sugar pine. The room can easily seat a thousand. Its 60-foot high ceiling, all of wood held together by pegs, was for many years the largest pillarless room in the United States. The enormous crown-shaped chandeliers, the damask wall covers, the rich carpeting, and other turn-of-the-century appointments make it one of the world's most elegant rooms.

Dine in the **Coronet Room** or the **Prince of Wales Grille,** then after dinner look into the Grand Ballroom overlooking the ocean. Roll out onto the courtyard to enjoy the colored lights and fountains.

As you drive down Coronado's quiet streets to the bridge, you'll glimpse the lights of San Diego. The skyline and its reflection dancing on the water will come into full view as you follow the curve of the bridge back to the city and follow the shoreline to your hotel.

# TOUR 3

### WHAT YOU'LL DO

- Breakfast at Casa Pedrorena in Old Town.
- Self-tour Old Town, with lunch and shopping at Bazaar del Mundo.
- Visit Sea World to see aquatic animal shows and ride the revolving tower capsule.
- Dine at Boom Trenchard's Flare Path.

### HOW YOU'LL DO IT

- Cab from hotel to Old Town's Pedrorena house, 2616 San Diego Avenue in Old Town; enter from Congress Street.
- Self-tour of Old Town's Seeley Stables, Casa de Estudillo, Historical Museum of Old California, the Bazaar del Mundo with lunch at Hamburguesa, 4016 Wallace Street.
- Cab from Old Town to Sea World, Mission Bay.
- Self-tour and guided tour of Sea World.
- Cab from Sea World to Boom Trenchard's, 2888 Pacific Coast Highway.
- Cab from restaurant to hotel.

### THINGS TO KNOW

- Casa de Pedrorena open 8:30 A.M.–9:30 P.M. daily. Since the area is closed to auto traffic, the cab will let you out a half block from the restaurant's rear entrance, which is accessible.
- Seeley Stables open 10:00 A.M.–6:00 P.M.; shows in theater at 11:00 A.M., 1:00 and 3:00 P.M. Admission 50¢ (ticket includes admission to Casa de Estudillo).
- Casa de Estudillo open 10:00 A.M. to 5:00 P.M. Two steps at door, but park ranger will open side door for level access.
- Sea World open 9:30 A.M. to dusk daily. Admission $5.50/ $3.25; rides 75¢/50¢.
- Boom Trenchard's serves dinner from 5:00 'til 2:00 A.M. Reservations advised.

$___/$___ indicates adult/child admission fees.
† All sites listed under "Restrooms" offer accessible facilities with wide stall doors and grab bars unless otherwise indicated.

RESTROOMS †

- Old Town, public area south of Plaza on Congress Street
- Hamburguesa
- Sea World

Probably nowhere else are California's early days of Mexican and American rule better or more extensively preserved than in **Old Town San Diego.** Named a state historic park in 1969, the six-and-a-half-block settlement offers a broad look at life in the 1829 to 1869 period.

Casa de Estudillo, a restored adobe home built around a lush courtyard, the original Seeley & Wright Stage Line terminal, and a town plaza of old trees are but the highpoints. Also to be seen are Yankee-style wood frame and brick houses, a former hacienda transformed into a bazaar of shops and restaurants, an adobe chapel, and a nineteenth-century hotel.

Unlike other old settlements that change with time, much of Old Town San Diego is as it was in the mid-nineteenth century. That's due to a shift in the economic and administrative focus of San Diego from the original settlement to a New Town built at the edge of her waterfront in the 1860s. Because Old Town buildings did not have to expand with the growth of the city, they remained as they were—to be rediscovered again in recent times.

What comes through for the visitor to Old Town is a sense that the nineteenth-century inhabitants have departed only moments before. This realness that one senses is intensified by the artful way the historic landmarks and museums are brought to life.

Begin your exploration of this early California world with pastry and coffee at the charming **Casa de Pedrorena.** The last of the adobes built in Old Town, it now houses a Mexican bakery and restaurant. Racks of freshly baked pastries dominate the front shop. Offerings seem to change minute by minute, but you'll probably find pumpkin bread, blueberry-filled *cuernos,* pink coconut cookies, and paper-thin crispy cookies. You can enjoy your selection among the weeping willow trees, pots of flowers and cactus in the lovely courtyard. Ask the waitress to bring coffee or tea, if you wish.

Continue with a visit to the reconstructed **Seeley Stable,** once a stagecoach terminal, now a museum of early conveyances and Western artifacts.

The accessible exhibits on the first floor include a recreation of a stable hand's room, the stage stop dining room, and an extensive display of vehicles. Old conveyances range from a royal Viennese carriage and elegant hearse to buggies and mud wagons. You can almost hear the clopping hooves on a country road as you see a buggie, shined gleaming for a picnic outing, complete with ribboned bonnet and food-filled hamper on its upholstered seats. A twenty-minute slide presentation tells the story of the growth of the transportation industry through the viewpoints of such historical characters as Father Serra, Black Bart, and Mark Twain.

For an interesting look at a scale model of Old Town as it was in the 1870s, bear to the left as you leave the Seeley Stable and continue to the **Historical Museum of Old California.** Then wheel along the path beside the building to San Diego Avenue. Along this historic main street you'll see a number of historic buildings, including Number 2645, which houses the **State Park Visitor's Information Center.** You can pick up a map and other materials here and make arrangements for a ranger to let you into the level side entrance of Casa de Estudillo.

If you have to wait for the ranger, tell the people at the information desk you'll be waiting in the **town plaza.** The lovely old plaza, across from the Casa de Estudillo, was the center of life in the old city. Sit under the same Portuguese cork and eucalyptus trees under which Mexican soldiers courted señoritas, and where sailors from trade ships and ranchers and merchants gathered to watch bull and bear fights. The cupola atop the Casa de Estudillo enabled the family within to watch the unending activity on this plaza.

Seeing the **Casa de Estudillo** may be the highlight of your visit to Old Town. The beautifully restored *casa* is built around an inner courtyard with orange calla and banana palm trees circling its blue tile fountain. As you roll along the terrace, you can look into many of the rooms. Coals in the brazier glow, candles flicker, and bowls of fresh fruit and flowers brighten the rooms, giving the impression that the family will return any moment. The furnishings represent what people of the Estudillo's class might have owned, and include such unusual items as an elegant Steinway piano, Blue Willow ware, a sixteenth-century monastic table, a grand American Empire rosewood bed. Note the lovely dining room with its Sheraton buffet, fine Mexican dining table, and a collection of silverware on the wall.

At the colorful **Bazaar del Mundo** across the the town plaza, you'll have the chance to taste food such as may have been served in the Casa de Estudillo. Located in the reconstructed Casa de Pico Hacienda, Bazaar del Mundo is a modern version of the market places of Mexico. The inner courtyard, complete with bandstand, is bordered by hibiscus and palm trees. Birds chirp in wrought iron cages. Bells tinkle in the breeze, and colorful banners flutter.

You can enjoy the garden scene from the outdoor **Casa de Pico** restaurant, choosing from a classic Mexican menu, or enter the charming **Hamburguesa Restaurant,** which features sixteen versions of hamburgers, steaks, salads, and desserts.

After lunch you'll want to tour the twenty shops that make up the bazaar, stopping to see the exotic potted plants at **The Plant Man,** the handicrafts and textiles from South America at **Tienda Panamericana,** and the original paintings at **The Gallery.**

Although you've only seen a portion of the twenty historic landmarks and places, the eight museums, twenty-five shops, and twelve restaurants within Old Town, you probably have seen the best of the accessible sights. If you're ready to move on, go by taxicab to Sea World.

You could easily spend all day at **Sea World,** with its six shows, thirty special exhibits, and three aquariums. But if you lunch early and get there by 1:00 P.M., you'll have a good five hours to see the highlights.

For those who don't have a lifetime to sail the seas of the world patiently peering through binoculars and hoping for a lucky break, Sea World provides a half-day alternative. In the time it takes to cover the eighty-acre marine-life showcase, you can see killer whales, white sharks, dolphins, penguins, seals, sea lions, otters, walruses, and hundreds of exotic fish from oceans throughout the world.

The real genius of Sea World is the way the animals are displayed. Some show off learned behaviors in entertaining themed shows. Others live in kelp beds, simulated Antarctic habitats, coral reef beds, or rocky tidal pools. Some of these are seen through windows, but others can be enjoyed from the series of open-air lagoons, ponds, and pools that dot the Sea World landscape.

Highlight for most is seeing Shamu, the three-ton killer whale who stars in his own show. Among his big acts is his newly learned "let's take the trainer for a ride." The harrowing ride begins as the trainer, mounted on the whale's slippery back and holding on for dear life, dives with the whale twenty-eight feet under the water. The act concludes as whale and trainer shoot twelve feet above the water and hit the surface with a resounding splash.

More amusing than harrowing are the antics of "the brainy bunch," dolphins that perform several times a day at a special dolphin arena. These intelligent creatures perform a wide-ranging series of back flips, mid-air spins, loops, and dives. One of their newest acts involves unusual team effort as three dolphins become a single surfboard that two trainers ride in tandem across the lagoon.

As thrilling as the shows are, the real joy of a visit to Sea World is getting to know its inhabitants at close range. Huge friendly walruses, smiling dolphins, and playful seals wait to be patted, hugged, or fed. Since more than 145 different kinds of birds and water fowl live in the ponds and gardens of Sea World, you also run into more than a few feathered friends. Doves perch on your shoulder, Igor the egret pokes his bill into your outstretched hand, Matilda the goose follows you, honking. Less impetuous are such rare birds as the magpie goose, harlequin duck, Jankowski's swan, and Abyssinian yellow-billed duck. As you roll between exhibits and shows over the beautifully maintained grounds, you can under-stand why many a winged freeloader swoops down to take a look at Sea World and stays on.

Sea World has won several awards for the most beautifully maintained recreation park gardens in the United States. A crew of twenty full-time gardeners care for the five hundred species of plants that now flourish on this former salt marsh. Annuals like poinsettias, cyclamen, primroses, pansies, and violas add color to a background of more subtle but rare Senegal date palms, succulents, endemic Torry pines, sago palms, and a large, authentically Japa-nese garden.

The lush flamingo pond may be the park's triumph. Stop to enjoy it, and then head for the unique new play environment called Cap'n Kids World. Designed to give youngsters the opportunity to express creativity, imagination, and sociability, the playground is one of only three of its kind in the world. Watch the youngsters climbing colored slopes of vinyl, bouncing on a giant air mattress, diving into a pool of 45,000 plastic balls, swinging over water, and climbing the fish net that leads to the Cap'n's Crows Nest.

You'll get a fine overview of the entire Sea World complex in the revolving capsule that travels up a 320-foot spire. The accessible ride provides a superb 360-degree view of Sea World, Mission Bay, and the city with its bay and hills.

If you leave Sea World just before it closes at dusk, your ride back to your hotel should provide lovely twilight views of water and hills. For dinner you can choose from the several accessible restaurants in the area where you're staying, or make a special outing to the unforgettable **Boom Trenchard's Flare Path Restaurant.** Combining aviation history with enticing entrees, the six-level restaurant is a flying buff's dream come true. Although only the first level is accessible, you'll see a life-size wooden statue of the Red Baron and his dog, Moritz, in the entry foyer, and a full-scale model of Otto Lilienthal's glider soaring overhead. At your table you'll get an unrestricted view of the flight operation at Lindbergh Field. All this and steak, lobster, and prime rib, too.

## TOUR 4

WHAT YOU'LL DO

- Visit Balboa Park, with stops at such attractions as the Fine Arts Gallery, Museum of Natural History, Timken Art Gallery, Museum of Man. Then lunch at the Cafe del Rey Moro (closed Mondays) and an organ concert.
- \* • Visit to the cottages of the House of Pacific Relations for open house entertainment and food.
- Dine at the Little America Westgate Hotel.
- Attend a concert or play at the Civic Theater.

\* Indicates restriction in time of visit.
$ /$ indicates adult/child admission fees.
† All sites listed under "Restrooms" offer accessible facilities with wide stall doors and grab bars unless otherwise indicated.

HOW YOU'LL DO IT

- Cab from your hotel to Balboa Park's Plaza de Panama.
- Push from Plaza area to Organ Pavilion.
- Push from Pavilion one-and-a-half blocks to House of Pacific Relations.
- Cab from House of Pacific Relations to hotel.
- Cab from hotel to Westgate Hotel.
- Push from Westgate Hotel to Civic Theater across street, 2nd and B streets.
- Cab from Civic Theater or Westgate Hotel to your hotel.

THINGS TO KNOW

- Balboa Park attractions open 9:00 A.M.–4:30 P.M. daily. Timken Gallery closed in September. Admission free except for Museum of Man 75¢/25¢; Natural History Museum admission $1.
- Cafe del Rey Moro luncheon served 11:00 A.M.–4:30 P.M., dinner 5:00–8:00 P.M., Tuesday thru Sunday. Enter from House of Hospitality, 1549 El Prado.
* • House of Pacific Relations open Sunday afternoons. Free.
- Westgate Hotel dining rooms: Westgate Room open 7:00 A.M.–11:30 P.M. daily; the formal Fontainebleau Room open 6:00 P.M.–10:30 P.M., 'til 11:00 P.M. on Friday and Saturday, closed Sunday.
- San Diego Civic Theater has wheelchair section in Dress Circle.

RESTROOMS †

- Fine Arts Gallery
- Casa del Prado Theater (off lobby)
- Westgate Hotel
- Civic Theater

You enter the seventeenth-century walled Spanish town via a graceful, arched bridge. The sense that you are discovering Spain in California grows as you see a reproduction of the ornate Mexico City Cathedral, and gardens that mirror those at Seville's Alcazar Castle. Beyond are a recreation of the rococo Hospital of Santa

Cruze de Toledo, the Basilica de Guadalupe, the town hall of Palma de Majorca, and the formal gardens of the Rhoda Palace.

You roll along the broad El Prado main boulevard, lined with a wealth of wood and plaster reminders of the 1915–16 Panama-California Exposition that celebrated the opening of the Panama Canal. Some of the temporary Spanish-Moorish style buildings have crumbled with the years and been replaced with exact duplicates.

The one-hundred-year-old **Balboa Park** got a major boost when it hosted the 1915–16 Panama-California Exposition and the California-Pacific International Exposition of 1935–36. The remnants and replacements from those eras today house a wealth of museums, theaters, halls, and restaurants.

You can easily spend the entire day exploring the heart of the 1400-acre park, choosing between visits to a dozen attractions, almost all of which are accessible, including five museums and art galleries, the lily pond and botanical display, and the English and Spanish gardens. You'll also need time to hear the world's largest outdoor organ at a special Sunday afternoon concert, lunch on the patio of the charming Cafe del Moro, and visit the House of Pacific Relations.

The **House of Pacific Relations** is a complex of fifteen cottages furnished in the style of a specific country. Every Sunday from 2:00 to 5:00 P.M. each cottage, staffed by local San Diegans in the dress of their ancestors, holds open house. The scene is one of great charm and warmth as the doors of the blue-shuttered houses open to reveal authentically furnished rooms, cabinets filled with china, tables covered in white lace. You are invited in to sip coffee or punch, to sample homemade cookies, cakes, and breads. In addition to the main program staged on the lawn, each house offers some of its own entertainment—a piano, or accordion player and singers.

On arrival get a map at the House of Hospitality located on the southeast corner of the main Panama de Pacific Plaza.

Note that the House of Pacific Relations is somewhat apart from the remainder of the park attractions. You may want to plan on visiting it last, leaving by cab from that location rather than wheeling back to the heart of the park attractions. If so, the ideal plan might be to attend the concert in the Spreckels Organ Pavilion at 2:00 P.M., then roll from the Pavilion to the House of Pacific Relations. This also happens to be the best route, considering curb cuts and traffic.

So with several hours to explore the park attractions, the problem becomes which ones to explore. If you have special interests such as flowers, art, natural history, or anthropology, your choices get easier. Should you simply like everything, then you'll have to try to see it all, concentrating on the following highlights:

At the **Museum of Man,** devoted to the anthropology and archeology of the American Indian cultures, see a pueblo and Aztec and Mayan ruins; watch Indians weave on handmade looms or grind acorns into flour with mortar and pestle.

Within the cool marble halls of the jewel-box **Timken Gallery,** see the beautiful collection of Russian icons and the Spanish, Dutch, and Flemish Renaissance paintings.

Under the redwood lattice of the **Botanical Building,** revel in the lush display of ferns and tropical blooms set under fifty-foot-tall palms.

At the **Museum of Natural History,** concentrate on the new Sefton Hall of Shore Ecology, which includes a film of California grunion breeding and a display of a tidal community at low and high tides.

In the **Fine Arts Gallery,** noted for its permanent collection of Old Masters and Asiatic art, see the first floor exhibit of impressionists' paintings.

If you missed visiting the Reuben H. Fleet Space Theater and Science Center on your outing to Balboa Park (see Tour 1 itinerary), you'll want at least to experience the revolutionary theater-planetarium show. Do it now.

At 2:00 P.M. an organist sits down before the world's largest outdoor organ at the **Spreckels Organ Pavilion** to continue a tradition of free Sunday concerts that began in 1915. Enjoy the sounds of the 3500-pipe masterpiece, then roll to the right of the organ and then west to the House of Pacific Relations. By the time you arrive, the costumed singers and dancers should be at their lively best.

From the folksy Europe you may have discovered at the House of Pacific Relations, you can enter the elegant Europe of kings and palaces. Remarkably enough, San Diego boasts one of the most elegant edifices this side of Versailles. It's the incomparable **Little America Westgate Hotel,** described by *Holiday* magazine's late Richard Joseph as one of the three greatest hotels in the world. Built at a cost of $15 million, the 235-room hotel is one man's Taj Mahal, a palace to beauty with little priority given to its economic sense. Here you can enjoy the wonder of public rooms filled with Aubusson and Beauvais tapestries, original Gainsborough and Fragonard oil paintings, Baccarat crystal chandeliers, and antiques. Among the latter is a $150,000 eighteenth-century marble fireplace, a $50,000 rosewood bombe commode signed by Linke, and a Henri Dasson desk worth $25,000. The parquet floor pattern is copied from those at Fontainebleau.

Stop for a drink in the **Plaza Bar,** where a pianist entertains on one of three gorgeous rosewood grand pianos. For dinner you can sample what the hotel calls "genteel American cooking" at the elegant but not imposing **Westgate Room.** On any day but Sunday, a second hotel dining option is the formal **Fontainebleau Room,** one of the most lavishly decorated rooms in America.

After dinner wheel across the street to the ultramodern **Convention and Performing Arts Center.** The totally accessible complex includes the stunning Civic Theatre, a plush 3000-seat arena that is acoustically perfect. It is hoped that you'll be attending a performance and can see the 10,000-crystal chandelier lit and dazzling.

### Other Accessible Attractions

Aerospace Museum, Ford Building, Balboa Park
Casa de Lopez Candle Shop
Mission San Diego de Alcala
Whaley House (enter via rear emergency exit door)
Cassius Carter Theatre (enter via Village Place service road)
Coronado Playhouse
Old Globe Theatre (enter via Village Place service road)
San Diego International Sports Arena (use north entrance)
San Diego Stadium
Starlight Bowl

Heritage Park
Wild Animal Park
Balboa Park Club

INTRODUCING
*Rollin' On* advisers, wheelers Aulton and Marene Aulger

*Title:* Active in Wheelacade, Inc., Paralyzed Veterans of America, the California Assn. of Physically Handicapped, Disabled Students Union, etc.
*Telephone number:* (714) 582–7648
*Hometown:* San Diego
*Favorite tourist site:* Reuben H. Fleet Space Theater and Museum
*Hidden corner:* Mickey Finn's
*Rendezvous:* Chief's Club, Naval Station
*Offbeat restaurant:* Pinnacle Peak in El Cajon
*Place for music:* Civic Theater
*View:* from the tip of Point Loma
*Natural wonder:* Mount Helix
*Museum:* Museum of Man
*Ramble:* out the Crystal Pier at Pacific Beach
*Non-tourist destination:* wheelchair dancing at Sharpe Hospital
*Offbeat experience:* a visit to Tijuana, Mexico, just a few miles from San Diego
*Traditional restaurant:* Mr. 'A' or El Cortez Hotel's Sky Room
*Low-cost restaurant:* Caesar's
*Ice cream shop:* Farrell's Ice Cream Parlour
*Reading suggestion: San Diego Magazine*
*Place to get a wheelchair repaired:* Skinner's on University Ave.
*Tip on having a great time in San Diego:* Just follow your nose anywhere in San Diego to any one of a hundred interesting places.

# 11

# San Francisco

It's where you left your heart . . . or are about to.

That's because in this city something magical happens. A mood creeps up to sweep you away. Without knowing when it happened, you're a kid again, ready simply to have fun, laugh, and enjoy the pleasures at hand.

In few cities will you find so many people with pleasure on their minds to keep you company. They've been called the gayest, lightest-hearted people anywhere. As they smile, speak, and wave, you'll find yourself responding. Before you know it, you'll be told of a new sight to see, know of a new restaurant to visit, or have a new friend. In few other cities will you find such a concentration of pleasures: beautiful views, lovely parks, good restaurants, abounding entertainment (even on street corners), rich museums, and artistic shops. As you roll and ride around the city finding the views you've seen in photos and the special places friends have told you about, you'll also find things no one told you about.

You'll see the streetcorner flower stalls, the sea lions at Seal Rock, the bay turn from blue to green to gray, the sloping hills of leafy trees and old Victorian houses.

You'll hear the fog horns, the street musicians, the sing-song strains of Oriental music in Chinatown, the clang and clatter of the cable cars.

You'll smell the salt air and fish at Fisherman's Wharf, the fragrance of green tea at the Japanese Tea Garden, the chocolate at Ghirardelli Square.

You'll taste sourdough French bread, fresh Dungeness crab, Irish coffee, and California Grey Riesling.

Then you'll find your own San Francisco as you come upon a hidden cafe with tiny trees and pots of tulips, a leafy park beside a skyscraper, or a view that encompasses purple bougainvillea, white sailboats, and blue sea.

You'll find the best, but when you leave San Francisco your heart will stay behind.

## Planning Your Trip

Aside from summer, when the city is very crowded, any time is a good time to visit San Francisco. You may run into rainy or foggy days any time of the year, however, but the fog can create a special mood, and as for rain, there's no way to figure when it will or won't occur.

Deciding when to come then will rest on your particular interests. If you'd like to be in town to hear the famous San Francisco Symphony Orchestra, then it must be between December and May. In May you can attend the Dollar Opera, sponsored by the Western Opera Theater at the Palace of Fine Arts. The cherry trees usually bloom in the Japanese Tea Garden at the end of March, and the rhododendrons in Golden Gate Park are at their peak in late April. The biggest art show is the one held each September at Civic Center plaza—it's the San Francisco Municipal Outdoor Art Festival. In December comes the Dicken's Christmas Faire held in the accessible Cow Palace.

If boats are your thing, and even if they're not, the Master Mariners' Regatta on San Francisco Bay on Memorial Day Weekend is a spectacle not to be forgotten.

To get information on these events and other helpful brochures and maps, write to the San Francisco Convention and Visitors Bureau, 1390 Market Street, San Francisco, California 94102. The Bureau puts out a listing of coming events that includes a key referring you to the appropriate box office that you can call or write to for price information and reservations.

For the current copy of *Guide to San Francisco for the Disabled*, send your request to the Easter Seal Society for Crippled Children and Adults, 6221 Geary Boulevard, San Francisco, California 94121.

## How to Get There

San Francisco is served by major airlines, Greyhound Lines, and Amtrak, which terminates at the Oakland Railroad Station. The San Francisco International Airport, about fifteen miles south of the city, is among the country's most accessible airports. In addition to what may be a perfect network of curb cuts, ramps and elevators, the airport also offers special transportation to other airport buildings, accessible restaurants, restrooms and even lowered telephones complete with amplifier and operating instructions in raised lettering. A brochure on the facilities for disabled persons may be obtained by writing to Airports Commission, San Francisco International Airport, San Francisco, California, 94128.

The Greyhound Terminal at 7th Street near Market Street is level, but restrooms are inaccessible.

## Getting Around

With its famous hills and Victorian vintage architecture, San Francisco on first look would seem to offer little to the wheelchair traveler. But on second look we discover that many of the tourist attractions lie in the flat areas encircling the hills. By knowing how to approach the attraction and which part to see, you can enjoy visits to Fisherman's Wharf, Chinatown, Embarcadero Center, Golden Gate Park, Union Street, Market Street, and Jackson Square.

Many of these areas now offer ramped crosswalks, thanks to the efforts of the Coalition for the Removal of Architectural Barriers (CRAB). This local group of disabled people and organizations was formed in 1974. Their first project was to get the city to cut all the curbs in the commercial centers, which includes the main tourist spots. They prepared a plan for ramps, made a proposal to the Public Works Department, and then got the city to commit itself to a five-year program to accomplish the task. Under the plan, 2500 curbs will be ramped by 1982. Already the ramps are completed along Market Street, at Fisherman's Wharf, in parts of Chinatown, and in the Embarcadero Center.

With 100 percent success on the first project, CRAB is on to their next one: lifts or platforms for wheelchair access to street cars. As one CRAB spokesman said, with typical California activism, "We won't stop until all buses are accessible and the handicapped no longer are confined to automobiles."

Already providing barrier-free rapid rail transportation within the city and beyond it to eighteen other communities is the Bay Area Rapid Transit system (BART). The system was constructed in compliance with the American National Standard Institute and with the advice of a Task Force on Handicapped Access. The result is that platform levels at each of the thirty-four stations are connected to street levels by elevators that have wheelchair-height controls and telephones. Passenger cars are also designed for wheelchair egress, with wide door openings, wide aisles, and only narrow gaps between the platform and car floor. Every BART station offers a restroom equipped for wheelchair users.

For the wheelchair traveler, BART opens up a world of sightseeing in San Francisco. Most popular are the stops at Civic Center, Powell Street, and the Embarcadero, with their adjacent attractions. Although Berkeley is twelve miles outside the city, most wheelers want to see it for its fame as America's most accessible city. You can get from the Embarcadero station to downtown Berkeley in nineteen minutes on BART.

BART also serves as a viewpoint for panoramas of the Bay and city. *Rollin' On* adviser John Edmonds suggests taking a sightseeing ride on BART to the Rockridge or Lafayette stations. When you arrive at either station, disembark onto the platform and catch the next train back to San Francisco. By not leaving the station you enjoy a long, beautiful ride for the minimum fare.

In addition to BART, San Francisco's taxicabs provide another means of getting around, particularly up and over the hills, which offer spectacular views. Because the distances are relatively short the high cab rates may not affect you or your wallet severely. Ferry boats also offer a unique means of getting around. By carefully scheduling your day, you can leave from the Ferry Building for a trip to Tiburon and return to San Francisco at the ferry's Fisherman's Wharf dock.

The three major car rental agencies rent vehicles with hand controls.

## Where to Stay

To really take advantage of BART and the inexpensive sightseeing it makes possible, you'll want to stay as close as possible to one of its stations. Several hotels, which are also accessible, are within a few feet of Bart.

The **Hyatt Regency,** 5 Embarcadero Center, is expensive, but you may find its convenience, amenities, and free evening entertainment worth the extra money you'll spend on a room.

Said to have the most spacious interior in America—excepting only Grand Central Station in New York—the hotel's atrium lobby stretches the length of a football field and rises seventeen stories. It has been the site for performances by the San Francisco Symphony Orchestra and the ballet—and for a goat milking contest sponsored by the 4-H, and a tightrope spectacle by a circus daredevil who crossed the lobby 200 feet in the air with no safety nets beneath.

Within this glass-roofed city, ivy cascades from balconies, a reflecting pool, fountain, and brook splash and babble, live birds sing, and lights twinkle in hundreds of ficus trees. More lights glitter in the five glass-enclosed elevators that rise from the lobby to a rooftop revolving lounge.

You'll enjoy the spectacle of this busy lobby, where people stroll as if they were in a park. By following the smoothly tiled promenade, you can join them windowshopping at the many shops, visiting the cafes and restaurants, and admiring the unusual art works, including a kinetic sculpture that imitates bird calls.

The lobby comes alive with the sound of music each afternoon and evening when a haunting instrument that is part reed and part piano is played and musicians stroll playing violins. Every Saturday the hotel puts on jazz concerts in the lobby and on Friday evenings a sixteen-piece band plays during a revival of the popular 1930s custom of tea dancing.

The hotel is totally accessible, with nine especially designed rooms for wheelchair visitors. In addition to its nearness to the Embarcadero Center BART station, the hotel is ideally situated for self-pushing. If you can manage an occasional uncut curb, you'll be able to go on your own to the plaza behind the hotel. There you'll see the controversial Vaillancourt Fountain, the five-block Embarcadero Center shopping-restaurant complex of which the hotel is part, and the Ferry Building, where you can board a boat bound for Tiburon, Sausalito, or Larkspur.

The **Holiday Inn-Civic Center,** 50 8th Street, is a half block off Market and within a full block of the BART Civic Center station. This functional, efficient hotel, with two rooms especially designed for paraplegics, is among the least expensive.

The **PSA San Franciscan Hotel,** 1231 Market Street, is across the street from the BART Civic Center station. With down-to-earth rates and great old world charm, it's a dream. Although the rooms were not specifically designed for wheelchair use, in 1976 the hotel met with leaders from the disabled community, seeking advice on how to bring rooms up to accessibility standards. Since the hotel is old, built in 1911, the rooms are spacious with wide doors, originally designed so that ladies in long full skirts could move in and out easily.

For many years the hotel, previously called the Whitcomb Hotel, was considered the finest hostelry west of the Mississippi. Today you see the remnants of the era when the hotel was San Francisco's glory. The flamboyant lobby boasts marble floors and colonnades, crystal chandeliers, an ornamental ceiling, huge beveled glass doors, and six $20,000 Tiffany domes. One dome glorifies the elegant Beppino's Italian restaurant, which is off the lobby.

By staying at the Holiday Inn–Civic Center or the PSA San Franciscan you'll not only have ready access to BART but also to the Orpheum Theater and Civic Auditorium, which both feature big name stars and musical groups. With some energy or assistance, you'll also be able to wheel over to the Opera House, Veteran's Auditorium, and the San Francisco Museum of Modern Art. Although this Market Street area presently boasts no great restaurants (with the exception of Beppino's in the PSA Hotel), it's the fastest growing part of San Francisco, and that picture is changing.

Although not near the BART stations, these are among the other hotels with rooms especially designed for wheelchair use:

TraveLodge at the Wharf, 250 Beach Street
Holiday Inn–Fisherman's Wharf, 1300 Columbus Avenue
Ramada Inn–Fisherman's Wharf, 590 Bay Stret
Sheraton at Fisherman's Wharf, 2500 Mason Street
Sheraton–San Francisco Airport, 1177 Airport Boulevard

## What You'll See and Do

Via BART, rented car, taxicab and wheelpower, you'll see the major sights, museums, parks, special neighborhoods and ethnic centers, and famous shopping complexes. But because San Francisco is a place where pleasure reigns, the tastebuds will be especially catered to. You'll find more reasons to stop for a sip or a nibble here than in any other city. Maybe it's the salty air. There'll be some new dishes to try, a new setting to experience, a view to savor, a sunny garden corner that invites you in. With any luck at all, you'll forget about sightseeing and settle down as the natives do simply to enjoy the good company, ambience, and views the city serves up.

With such possibilities in mind, the majority of suggested itineraries are minitours to be enjoyed in a morning or afternoon. All trips except one use BART or taxicabs. The final full-day itinerary, because of the distance it covers, makes the use of a car necessary.

### Among the Accessible Restaurants

American
Assay Office, 56 Gold Street
Grand Exhibition, Sheraton at Fisherman's Wharf
The Hippo, Van Ness at Pacific
House of Prime Rib, 1906 Van Ness Avenue
Iron Duke, 132 Bush Street
Mac Arthur Park, 607 Front Street
Market Place, Hyatt Regency
Monte Jusco's Caffe, 2333 Powell Street
Perry's, 1944 Union Street

Salmagundi, 355 Bush Street, 442 Geary, 2 Embarcadero
Center
Tommy's Joynt, Geary at Van Ness Avenue
What This Country Needs Restaurant, 1st and Market streets
Vista Cafe, 2765 Hyde Street
Zim's, Northpoint Shopping Center, Bay at Mason streets

## Chinese
Empress of China, 838 Grant Avenue
Far East Cafe, 631 Grant Avenue
Mandarin, Ghirardelli Square
Shang Yuen, The Cannery

## Continental
Adolph's, 641 Vallejo Street
Bardelli's, 243 O'Farrell Street
Carnelian Room, Bank of America Building
Henry's Fashion, 252 California Street
Hugo's, Hyatt Regency Hotel

## English
Ben Jonson, The Cannery

## French
Ernie's, 847 Montgomery Street
Jack's, 615 Sacramento Street
Old Brittany, The Cannery

## German
Schroeder's, 240 Front Street (steep ramp)

## Indian
Anjuli, One Embarcadero Center (enter via Battery Street)
India House, 350 Jackson Street

## International
Magic Pan, Ghirardelli Square
Paprikas Fono, Ghirardelli Square

## Italian
Beppino's Ristorante, PSA San Franciscan Hotel
Caesar's, 2299 Powell Street
Fior d'Italia, 621 Union Street

Green Valley, 510 Green Street
La Pantera, 1234 Grant Avenue
North Beach Restaurant, 1512 Stockton Street
Veneto, 389 Bay Street

Japanese
Fujiya, One Embarcadero Center

Mexican
El Sombrero, The Cannery
La Cucina, 2136 Union Street
Widow and Pancho Villa, 470 Pacific Avenue

Seafood
Castagnola, Jefferson and Jones
Hungry Tiger, The Cannery
Scoma's, Pier 47 behind Pompeii's Grotto (several steps at entrance, but very helpful personnel)
Sinbad's Pier 2, Embarcadero at Mission Street

Skyrooms
Carnelian Room, 555 California Street
Equinox, Hyatt Regency Hotel
Fairmont Crown, Fairmont Hotel
Top of the Mark, Mark Hopkins Hotel
Veranda Lounge, Holiday Inn–Union Square

You'll find other possibilities in the restaurant listing put out by the Convention and Visitors Bureau, in *Key*, *Where*, and *San Francisco* magazine; call for information.

Should you have some time for meeting other wheelers during your visit, the Indoor Sports Club is a lively group, sometimes holding evening coffee get-togethers in San Francisco. For information, call Russ Bohlke at 823–7270.

If special questions relating to accessibility or getting around in general come up, a good source for information is the California Association of Physically Handicapped (CAPH), a statewide organization of 3000 activists lobbying for the disabled. Call them in San Francisco at 543–CAPH (543–2274).

# MINITOUR 1

### WHAT YOU'LL DO

- Tour and shop in Chinatown.
- Visit the Chinese of China Restaurant.
- Lunch at the Empress of China Restaurant.
- Tour Jackson Square.
- Libation at a Gold Street restaurant.

### HOW YOU'LL DO IT

- Cab from hotel to corner of Jackson and Grant Avenue in the heart of Chinatown.
- Push four blocks down west side of Grant Avenue, then push three blocks up east side of Grant Avenue to Empress of China Restaurant, 838 Grant, sixth floor.
- Cab from Empress of China Restaurant to the corner of Jackson and Montgomery Street.
- Push one or two blocks, then stop at Assay Office restaurant, 56 Gold Street.
- Cab from Assay Office to hotel.

### THINGS TO KNOW

- Chinatown Wax Museum open 10:00 A.M.–11:00 P.M. daily; $1.50/$1.
- Empress of China serves lunch from 11:30 A.M.
- Assay Office open 11:30 A.M.–10:00 P.M.

### RESTROOMS †

* • Transamerica Pyramid (key available from fifth floor building office near elevator, weekdays only).

$___/$___ indicates adult/child admission fees.
† All sites listed under "Restrooms" offer accessible facilities with wide stall doors and grab bars unless otherwise indicated.

Separate and surprisingly exotic, San Francisco's **Chinatown** after 125 years remains an American Canton. The scene is out of Fu Manchu: calligraphy street signs, dragon-entwined lamp posts, filigreed balconies, a roofscape of arched eaves and pagodas. Ancient Chinese women in mandarin jackets and black trousers select ginger and bamboo shoots at neighborhood markets. Old men read Chinese newspapers posted outside print shops; sing-song strains of popular Oriental tunes drift from corner newsstands.

Since a good percentage of the 70,000 Chinese who live in San Francisco reside within this twenty-four-block settlement—the largest outside the Orient—Chinatown is not just a bazaar for tourists. It's where these Chinese-Americans market, bank, visit their doctors, dine out, see movies, and socialize. It's for real—the largest and most authentic glimpse of China you'll have this side of Hong Kong.

As you can imagine, Chinatown is a busy place. It also has narrow streets, which makes it wise to schedule your visit at its least hectic time—midmorning or midafternoon.

Since Grant Avenue slopes downhill from California Street to Jackson Street, have your cab driver let you off at the corner of California Street and Grant Avenue so you can roll down the four blocks to Jackson Street. If more energy or assistance comes your way, you can roll back up Grant Avenue on the opposite side of the street. Get out of the cab at the northwest corner of California Street and Grant Avenue at the **Chinatown Wax Museum.** Inside you'll see the China of Marco Polo and early California brought to life in thirty-one scenes inhabited by 115 figures created by master wax sculptors in Hong Kong. It's a fascinating history lesson and also brings into focus some of the exotic pictures that books may have created for you. You'll see early-day immigrants working on the first transcontinental railroad, in the California gold fields, Chinatown laundries, and fortune cookie factories.

Some of the early Chinatown attractions that you saw in wax still exist in living concrete, for example the **Bank of Canton** building at 743 Washington Street, which for many years was the special Chinatown telephone exchange. On the east side of Grant Avenue you'll see **Tin Bow Tong,** an old Chinese pharmacy and herb shop, at 947 Grant Avenue.

Now begin your tour, choosing the Bay or east side of Grant Avenue with its variety of shops, its bakery, and its access to the Trade Center and to the remarkable Empress of China Restaurant.

First you'll come to the **Eastern Bakery** where you can choose between the rice candy, black bean or lotus coconut cakes, and sesame or giant fortune cookies.

Across the street you'll find the **Ching Chong Company,** a grocery store with bins of strange-looking vegetables, and ducks hanging in the windows. Inside you probably can find 1000-year-old eggs, sharks' fins, dried seahorses, lichee nuts, and, happily, wonderful candied melon or ginger.

The **China Trade Center** at 838 Grant is a multilevel complex of shops accessible by elevator. Notice the golden dragon that winds around the staircase. On the basement level, look into **Chong Kee Jan Company** and see its Chinese cooking utensils, feather fans, silk lanterns, baskets, parasols, and tins of tea. If you roll to the back door, you can look out onto Portsmouth Square, where Chinatown's senior citizens sit in the sun and children play.

The **Empress of China Restaurant** on the sixth floor of the Center claims, in all humility, to have one of the most beautiful interiors in the world. A 30-foot temple built by Taiwan palace craftsmen has been reassembled here. Within it is a re-creation of the Dowager Queen's pleasure park in Peking. Small pine trees grow inside the temple, which is domed in ornamental glass, filled with flowers, and has fierce green dog statues guarding its treasures. Overlooking the temple or the roof garden, one can sample such specialties as lobster Canton, lichee chicken, 100-blossom lamb, barbecued quail, whole winter melon, North China onion bread, and flaming sweets.

An alternate to the luxurious Empress is the excellent **Far East Cafe,** on the opposite side of the street at 631 Grant Avenue.

After lunch continue your tour with a look inside the **Bank of Trade** at 1001 Grant, where you'll see interesting old Chinese furniture, antique check-writing stands, and abacuses for adding up checkbooks.

If you're serious about shopping, you can spend days in Chinatown, looking among the porcelain spoons and bowls, the huge carved smiling Buddhas, the mandarin-style clothing, the back scratchers, and bronze dragon paper weights. Most shops are on the street, with level access.

When you're ready to move on, wheel with assistance down Jackson Street two steep blocks to Montgomery Street, or take a cab the long way, up Grant Avenue and down Columbus Avenue with its colorful street life.

Before visiting historic **Jackson Square,** stop to enjoy the fountains and redwood trees in the little park behind the **TransAmerica Pyramid** at Montgomery and Washington streets. Then roll into the lobby for a look at the artwork exhibited on its walls, and take a ride to the twenty-seventh floor for a memorable view from this public observation area (weekdays only). Although curbs aren't ramped in this area of the city, you'll find a driveway on Washington Street that will allow you to roll along one side of Jackson Street, and then cross to a second alley that links with Gold Street. By doing this you'll have access to the most interesting sights within this four-square-block area.

Hitching posts, old brick buildings with iron shutters, and fine Federal-style facades take one back to the early days when Jackson Street was the heart of Gold Rush San Francisco. Wells Fargo coaches, hansom cabs, and drays clattered in and out of the livery stable on Hotaling Place. Miners from the Mother Lode dumped nuggets and gold dust onto the counters of Gold Street assayers' offices. The character of the old West remains, although it's a very polished old West indeed. Rolling past the renovated nineteenth-century buildings, you'll see some of the most alluring window displays in the West. The majority of shops specializing in interior decoration are open only to the wholesale trade, but you'll find some retail outlets, primarily those selling fine furnishings, antiques, and artifacts.

Of the thirty-seven buildings in the Jackson Square area, seventeen have been proclaimed landmarks. Note particularly the building at 472 Jackson, constructed in 1850 using ships' masts as interior supporting columns. If you have assistance, wheel around the corner to 722 Montgomery Street, where frock-coated gentlemen once attended musical revues at the Melodeon. The building now houses the showplace offices of attorney Melvin Belli.

On Gold Street you'll find several art galleries and the **Assay Office** restaurant. You might stop at the restaurant to get more of the flavor of the neighborhood, to marvel at the stained glass ceiling, and to do what the miners did when they came to town with parched throats.

## MINITOUR 2

WHAT YOU'LL DO

- Mid-afternoon visit to Union Street for look at shops and galleries; early dinner.
- Twilight drive along Marina Green and Yacht Harbor.
* • Visit to the Exploratorium at the Palace of Fine Arts.

HOW YOU'LL DO IT

- Cab from hotel to the Artists' Coop, 2224 Union Street.
- Push one to two blocks east on Union Street.
- Cab from Union Street restaurant via the Marina Green to the Palace of Fine Arts, Baker and Beach streets.
- Cab from Palace to hotel.

THINGS TO KNOW

- Union Street stores and restaurants open until 5:00 or 6:00 P.M.
* • Exploratorium open Wednesday evening 7:00–9:30 P.M., Wednesday–Sunday, 1:00–5:00 P.M. No admission fee, but donations encouraged.

RESTROOMS

- No wheelchair-accessible facilities available in vicinity.

* Indicates restriction in time of visit.

You'd have to wait forever for the cows to come home to San Francisco's old Cow Hollow. But although the cows are gone, some of the barns and dairies that dominated west **Union Street** in the 1800s remain. Renovated clapboard dwellings, carriage houses, barns, stables, and a dairy now house antique shops, florists, handicraft galleries, and cafes. Passages lead between buildings to flower-filled courtyards, Dutch doors and iron gates open onto garden cafes. Gas lamps flicker.

Although Union Street's curbs are high and at the moment unramped, you can, by being assisted over one set of corner curbs, see the choicest part of this charming street. Have your cab driver let you out at the **Artists' Cooperative,** which is owned by artists who display their own works and that of new talent. Drop in the spacious gallery to see the current one-man show and to look over the fine showing of graphics, stained glass, and sculpture.

From the Coop continue across the intersection at Fillmore, rolling to **Jurgensen's,** one of the most beautiful grocery stores in the country. Sniff the Maui onions, fresh sorrel, horseradish, fenugreek, and ginger, then sample a strawberry dipped in white chocolate, or a stuffed date—or both.

At **Trattoria Moresco's,** down the street, you'll see more beautiful food, this time in a deli where you can also buy Polish sausage, beef tongue sandwiches, mushroom turnovers, or soup. Little cafe tables with starched, blue-and-white checked table cloths and tiny vases of flowers invite repose. You'll be well situated for people-watching at a table near the window overlooking the busy street.

At the **Flower Boutique,** you'll come to an iron gate opening onto a walkway that leads between two buildings to a "secret" hidden garden. In this cool retreat of old trees, ferns, and potted flowers, you can stop to hear the birds singing and to watch the florist's playful cat. Take a look at the miniature topiaries and unusual dry flower arrangements inside the former stable that's now a workroom and shop.

With a little help getting up the slight incline that leads from the florist's shop to the street, you'll be on your way to the Victorian antique shop a door or two away. You'll know you have the right place when you see the shop owner's cat sleeping on a lace-covered pillow. Note the Victorian beadwork and china lamps, the old sterling ware, the period spelter pieces, the old stained glass, and perhaps a black lace umbrella.

If you're ready for lunch, a good choice is **La Cucina Restaurant,** with windows opening onto a garden. The sunlit restaurant serves classic dishes, including hamburgers, steaks, and cheeseboards with fruit.

You can continue your Union Street tour or take a cab from the restaurant after lunch to the **Exploratorium,** which is inside the monumental **Palace of Fine Arts.** The famous building, designed by

Bernard Maybeck for the city's 1915 Panama-Pacific International Exposition, reigns over a lagoon where ducks paddle. Ask your cab driver to approach the Palace so you can see something of this old Greco-Romanesque confection.

Roll into the science museum, which is more like an indoor public park than a conventional museum. The phenomena of nature are freely available in this three-acre cavern where the visitor chooses his own pathway to any of the four hundred displays designed to dramatize scientific principles. Parabolic sound mirrors, a momentum machine, the relative motion swing, and a sun painting invite you to examine your perceptual powers. Most of the exhibits are designed to be manipulated; for those who are uncertain, a museum guide or "explainer" especially trained to teach is usually nearby ready to show one how.

It's easy to get into the spirit of the museum as you touch, pound, open, pull on, look through, listen to, or yell at the unbelievable assortment of contraptions. You watch others involved in the exhibits, offer advice, ask questions, and laugh with them at the pleasure of discovery. You could spend hours at the Exploratorium, especially on a Wednesday evening, when informal concerts are often presented, followed by musician and audience discussions.

By planning your schedule carefully, you can go from the Exploratorium to a performance at the **Palace of Fine Arts Theater,** which is in the same building. You can remain in your chair in the accessible theater. Buy snacks before the performance from the gourmet concession stand.

## MINITOUR 3

WHAT YOU'LL DO

- Visit the San Francisco Maritime Museum.
- Enjoy the entertainment, lunch, and shops at Ghirardelli Square.

$___/$___ indicates adult/child admission fees.

† All sites listed under "Restrooms" offer accessible facilities with wide stall doors and grab bars unless otherwise indicated.

- Dine at The Cannery or take a ramble along Fisherman's Wharf and have dinner at a seafood restaurant.

### HOW YOU'LL DO IT

- Cab to the Maritime Museum, Polk and Beach streets.
- Push across street to Ghirardelli Square. Use street level elevators on Beach Street.
- Push through Victorian Park bordering Beach Street.
- Push, or with assistance go down Leavenworth Street one moderately steep hill to Jefferson Street and the level entranceway into The Cannery.
- Push one or two blocks to Fisherman's Wharf.
- Cab from The Cannery or a Wharf restaurant to your hotel.

### THINGS TO KNOW

- Maritime Museum open 10:00 A.M.–5:00 P.M. daily, $1/50¢.
- The Cannery and Ghirardelli Square shops and restaurants are open late. Dinner reservations advised.
- Concerts are frequent at The Cannery. Call to find out the schedule for the day.

### RESTROOMS †

- Maritime Museum (stalls 25 inches wide)
- Holiday Inn–Fisherman's Wharf, 1300 Columbus Avenue
- The Cannery and Ghirardelli Square (restrooms accessible, but stall less than 25 inches wide)

It's a festival of kids flying kites and vendors hawking balloons, of street people selling their wares and entertaining with music and dance. Drums beat, horns toot, guitars "take off," and cable cars clatter and jingle. Onto the scene comes a girl with a basket of flowers, a man in velvet cloak and plumed hat, an American Indian with his face painted, blacks with wild Afro hairstyles and bongo drums, a lady in a fur coat with a Japanese parasol.

You're in the scene at San Francisco's **Victorian Park,** a stretch of green lawn, gas lamps, and flower beds ringed by the city's greatest waterfront attractions. To the east the ship-shaped building that houses the Maritime Museum is at anchor above Aquatic Park. To the west lies The Cannery. To the south reigns the rococo

Ghirardelli Square. Northward stretches the bay, at different times surprisingly blue or bottle green or gray.

The order of your visit to Ghirardelli Square and The Cannery is important, since there's a steep hill between the two. By going to Ghirardelli Square first, you then can go down rather than up Hyde Street to the accessible Jefferson Street entrance of The Cannery.

Since the **Maritime Museum** is close to Ghirardelli Square, begin your tour with a stop there, entering via the door at the Senior Citizens Center on the east side of the Museum building. You'll be able to explore the first-floor exhibits, which focus on San Francisco's maritime history. Instead of only displaying ship models and paintings, however, the museum has turned the telescope around to focus on the physical mass of the great ships that once docked in the bay. Here you'll see real figureheads, wrought iron caps and truss bows, wheel pumps, a huge anchor, and the trailboards outlining the massive bow of a big lumber schooner. On the outdoor terrace overlooking Aquatic Park, you'll see the tiny vessel in which Kenichi Horie made his famous one-man voyage from Japan to San Francisco in 1962.

When you leave the museum, roll down Beach Street to the Beach Street arcade leading into Ghirardelli Square. An elevator will take you to the main plaza.

Recipient of a rarely bestowed American Institute of Architects medal, **Ghirardelli Square** is one of the first shopping-dining complexes utilizing renovated industrial buildings. This one uses the seventy-five-year-old Ghirardelli Chocolate Factory complex as centerpiece. The historic factory, a copy of the French Chateau Blois, is a gingerbread confection—dark red brick with cream-colored trim and complete with clock tower. Around the old buildings a labyrinth of terraces, plazas, and walkways serves as the stage for viewing the bay and links the beehive of eighty shops and cafes. Trees twinkling with lights, tubs of flowers, sculpture, an enchanting mermaid fountain, and colorful kiosks complete the scene. The information kiosk between the two plazas dispenses maps showing you how to find your way around the Cocoa, Mustard, Chocolate and Wurster buildings, and through the Clock Tower, Woolen Mill, and Power House.

Built to be wheelchair-accessible, you'll find six elevators and dozens of ramps to get you anyplace you'd like to go. But part of the adventure of exploring Ghirardelli Square is getting lost and seeing if you can find your way out without stopping for something to eat or drink in a newly discovered cafe or tavern. As you wheel around this two-and-a-half-block maze, you'll want to stop to hear the free entertainment presented off and on between 11:00 A.M. and 2:00 P.M. near the Mermaid Fountain. Also, look into the unusual **Come Fly a Kite** shop, with its kites from all over the world; the **Almond Plaza,** known to give away free samples; and the **Light Opera** gallery, with its art glass.

When it comes to food you can choose from the outdoor patio of the **Bratskellar,** the authentic **Indian Gaylord Restaurant,** the **Ghirardelli Wine Cellar** with monk-robed waiters, the country-style **Paprikas Fono Restaurant,** and a half dozen more. As the fragrance of chocolate lures you toward the **Ghirardelli Chocolate Manufactory** ice cream parlor, you can nicely rationalize your need to enter by knowing it's also a museum. As you look at the old chocolate machinery blending luscious dark chocolate, you may also catch sight of fudge-topped sundaes being served and, without further anguish, fittingly complete your visit to Ghirardelli Square with one of your own.

Continue from the Square along Beach Street to Hyde Street and with assistance take the steep incline down Hyde Street to Jefferson Street. At this intersection you'll see the **San Francisco Historic Ships Pier** with its four old California coastal vessels. Although the boats aren't accessible, you might find it worthwhile to wheel along the pier to inspect the three-masted lumber schooner, a steam schooner, a double-ended bay ferryboat, and a square-ended scow. You can hear what it was like (complete with crashing waves) when they were in their seagoing prime by listening to the audio-guide headset included in the price of admission.

Like a beautiful woman who wants to be loved for her mind **The Cannery** bids visitors to look beyond its pleasing exterior. There's something more than mere beauty to be discovered in this unique shopping-dining complex; for the discerning eye, there's an architecture that can only be called human. It is the result of the vision of its developer to create a totally effective people place, accomplished by facilitating the movement of people and at the same time exposing this movement so that the observer can see how spaces are connected. In this way people actually become part of the design. They move horizontally, vertically, and diagonally from terraces to arcades, up stairways and elevators, along a sloping glass-roofed escalator. This visible movement elicits participation. Without realizing it, one is suddenly part of a special community, a separate world within a walled city or an Italian galleria. You may join this world as you roll onto the central courtyard of The Cannery, seeing yourself—with only a little imagination—as one of a ballet troupe performing on stage.

Music helps performance, and there's usually plenty at The Cannery: a violin and guitar duo playing "Turkey in the Straw," a jazz saxophonist tooting "When the Saints Go Marchin' In," or a harpist rendering an old English folk song. Free entertainment is part of the scene, as are the performing magicians, mimes, jugglers, dancers, and puppeteers.

As you enjoy the entertainment you'll also be able to take a visual tour of the former peach canning factory. A hardy survivor of the 1906 earthquake and fire, this old Del Monte Cannery was redesigned and reconstructed in 1967 when a developer saw its potential as an urban center. The original red brick exterior with its arched windows was preserved, but the interior was redesigned. On the site where formerly a railway siding ran is the courtyard, with its old olive trees and flower carts. The old interior became a labyrinth of shops, galleries, restaurants, markets, and pubs.

You can see these on all three levels by riding the glass-enclosed elevator or a second elevator to the north. Not to be missed is The Cannery's Elizabethan pub and restaurant, **Ben Jonson's.** The restaurant is built around an authentic English gallery transplanted from Albyn's Hall in Stappleford Abbey, Essex; three Elizabethan dining rooms with fireplaces; and a seventeenth-century oak staircase. Brought to America in the 1920s by William Randolph Hearst, they were purchased by The Cannery's owner, Leonard Martin, and reassembled at the Ben Jonson.

The main floor dining room of Ben Jonson's is rich with Old English rugs and antiques. You can lunch on such specialties as "toad in the hole" (sausage wrapped in pastry), rarebit, or a cheeseboard with fruit—all served by "serving wenches" in appropriate old English costumes.

At **El Sombrero** next door, amidst an environment of cool Spanish tiles, wrought iron chandeliers, leather-wicker furniture, you can let your taste buds go south of the border. And at the **Old Brittany,** a charming French cafe with starched white curtains, you can try French onion soup, crêpes, truffles, and casseroles.

After sampling a restaurant, follow the zigzagging corridors to the fifty shops, stop to people-watch and enjoy the entertainment, then roll out the Jefferson Street entrance to be in the heart of Fisherman's Wharf. Jefferson Street is the busiest and most interesting of the Wharf streets, with its pots of steaming crab, loaves of French sourdough bread, curios, and, oh yes, fishing boats. Continuing a block or two, you'll come to a wharf where some of the sports fishing boats and tuna trawlers are tied up.

As you taxi back to your hotel from the Wharf, ask your driver to pass the *Balclutha*, anchored at Pier 43. Lights illuminate the tall masts of this, the last full-rigged ship of the great Cape Horn fleet. As you pass you may think you hear the "anchors aweigh" call and are about to see the fully-rigged vessel cast off on its historic course along the world's greatest nineteenth-century trade route.

## MINITOUR 4

WHAT YOU'LL DO

- Tour the Fairmont Hotel and have libations in the Fairmont Crown skyroom.
* • Attend the Sunday afternoon concert at Grace Cathedral.
- Sip and sightsee at twilight from the Top of the Mark.

HOW YOU'LL DO IT

- Cab from your hotel to Fairmont Hotel.
- Push three blocks to Grace Cathedral, bounded by California, Sacramento, Taylor and Jones streets; enter from Sacramento Street parking lot.

* Indicates restriction in time of visit.
† All sites listed under "Restrooms" offer accessible facilities with wide stall doors and grab bars unless otherwise indicated.

- Push three blocks to the Mark Hopkins Hotel, California at Mason Street.
- Cab from Mark Hopkins Hotel to your hotel.

THINGS TO KNOW

- Fairmont Crown room open 11:00 A.M.–2:00 A.M. daily for cocktails; Sunday brunch from 10:30 A.M.
* - Grace Cathedral concerts held most Sunday afternoons at 5:00 P.M. Phone Cathedral to double check.
- Top of the Mark open daily 10:00 A.M. to 2:00 A.M.

RESTROOMS †

- Grace Cathedral

Whenever a visitor sets out to see the city and environs from atop one of San Francisco's eleven skyrooms, he or she gambles at seeing nothing at all. That's because by the time one reaches the rooftop viewpoint, the city's famous fog can creep in "on little cat feet." But even fog watching has its charm. Gray billows descend in fantasy shapes, accenting the colors of the sunset or veiling the moon and stars with peek-a-boo caprice.

On clear days, however, windows open onto fifty-mile panoramas of bay, ocean, bridges, mountains, foothills, and skylines. Since one really wants to see both the daytime and twilight views, this day is planned to include both.

First you'll visit the **Fairmont Hotel,** a marble palace designed by Stanford White. The lobby is one of the most spacious around, with plush carpeting, velvet settees, high ceilings, and lots of marble, gilt, crystal, and mirrors. The adjacent twenty-nine-story Tower was added to the original seven-story heart of the hotel in 1961.

The most scenic way to reach the top of the Tower is via "the thermometer," a glass-enclosed elevator that glides up and down the tower's east face. Then from the spacious **Crown** you can enjoy the incredible 360-degree view while lunching or simply sipping.

Continuing from the hotel along California Street you'll pass the distinguished Pacific Union Club, built in 1885 by a "bonanza baron." The brass fence that encircles it used to be kept shining by a workman paid only to rub and buff the railings. Next to the Club lies the elegant little Huntington Park.

Since you'll be entering Grace Cathedral from Sacramento Street, wheel back along Mason Street to Sacramento. From this crest you'll get a different view as you look down to the bay. Then proceed along Sacramento past the charming townhouses to the Cathedral parking lot entrance.

**Grace Cathedral,** the largest gothic structure in the West, approximates Notre Dame. Buttresses ornamented with pinnacles, gargoyles, a cross finished in gold leaf, and a carillon of forty-four bells embellish the edifice. Inside you see a glory of stained glass: the great rose window above the main portal and windows with love, fortitude, peace, and astronauts as their subjects.

By going out one of the side doors at the main entrance of the Cathedral, you'll get a look at the golden doors that are replicas of those on Florence's Baptistry of San Giovanni. The two-ton double doors, made of bronze overlaid with gold, are composed of ten panels of Old Testament scenes. Detailing has been chased painstakingly; one craftsman spent six weeks detailing a postcard-sized section bringing out every feather on a bird. Ask for the pamphlet that gives the history of the doors and tells the biblical story of each of the panels.

Concerts are given many Sunday afternoons at 5:00 P.M. The programs can feature a single organist, the Cathedral Choir, a high school or college choir, a concert using all four of the Cathedral's organs, or Turk Murphy playing vespers. The Cathedral, among the most innovative in the country, is also the setting for programs featuring authentic Indian sitar music and showing films like *King of Kings* with live musical accompaniment.

After the concert push along California Street for your twilight date at the **Top of the Mark.** Although the main entrance is level, it has several stairs. So, if you have assistance, go a few feet down the steep California Street hill to the level entrance a few feet away. Should you need help, one wheeler reports that the doormen at the Mark "couldn't be more delightful and happy to help."

Built in 1926 by railroad tycoon Mark Hopkins, the hotel occupies the choicest site on Nob Hill. In 1939 the private penthouse on the nineteenth floor was converted into a cocktail lounge. Since then it's entertained almost 32 million visitors, including service-men who gave their farewell toast to the States from this room be-fore shipping out to the World War II battlegrounds in the Pacific.

Feel free to tour the room and enjoy its 360-degree view before choosing the ideal spot for sunset cocktails. If the fog horns are silent, your viewscape of bay, ocean, bridges, boats, hills, and can-yons will be painted pink by the setting sun. Its afterglow will dust the clouds with rosy light as the city lights shine in the gathering dusk.

## TOUR 1

WHAT YOU'LL DO

- Shop and lunch at Embarcadero Center.
* • See Vaillancourt Fountain, and shop among the street-vendor stalls.
* • Visit the Mines & Geology Museum weekdays in the Ferry Building.
- Cruise to Tiburon, with visits to waterfront shops and cafes.
- Dine at Fisherman's Wharf.

HOW YOU'LL DO IT

- Push from Embarcadero BART station to Embarcadero Cen-ter, Sacramento, Clay, Drumm, and Battery streets.
- Push two blocks to Justin Herman Plaza, Market at Embarca-dero Street.
- Push across street to Ferry Building, foot of Market Street.
- Push from Ferry Building to adjacent boat dock.
- Push along Tiburon's Main Street.
- Push from Fisherman's Wharf dock to restaurants and shops along Jefferson Street.
- Cab from Wharf to hotel.

THINGS TO KNOW

* • Vaillancourt Fountain's street merchants out during weekday lunch hours and early afternoon.

* Indicates restriction in time of visit.
† All sites listed under "Restrooms" offer accessible facilities with wide stall doors and grab bars unless otherwise indicated.

* • Mines & Geology Museum open weekdays, 9:00 A.M.–5:00 P.M.
 • Tiburon-bound ferries depart from the Ferry Building terminal only at 7:30 A.M. and 4:25, 5:15, 5:45, and 7:10 P.M. Call Harbor Carriers to check times—546–2815.
 • San Francisco-bound ferries that dock at Fisherman's Wharf depart from Tiburon at 5:00, 5:55, and 8:00 P.M.
 • Fisherman's Wharf restaurants open late. Reservations advised.

   RESTROOMS †

 • Hyatt Regency Hotel
 • Sabella's Restaurant, 9 Main Street, Tiburon
 • Sheraton at Fisherman's Wharf, 2500 Mason Street
 • Ramada Inn–Fisherman's Wharf, 590 Bay Street
 • Holiday Inn–Fisherman's Wharf, 1300 Columbus Avenue

Any kid will tell you that one of the main reasons for coming to San Francisco is so that you can ride a ferry boat. If you've been raring to taste the salt spray, hear the slapping waves, and get to know a sea gull in his own element, this is your day. Although you could choose from several cruises offered by Harbor Tours, maybe you'll find your sea voyage more memorable aboard one of the small cruisers that ferries the natives to and from Tiburon or Sausalito.

Wheelers say the trip to Tiburon is best because the shops and restaurants along the tiny village's Main Street are accessible—and there's also a restroom equipped for wheelchairs at one of the big restaurants. Whether you choose Tiburon, Sausalito, or both, you can board a ferry beside the Ferry Building (appropriately enough) and thus be in an interesting area beforehand for sightseeing and shopping. With some careful planning, you can board the ferry bound for Tiburon at the Ferry Building, but instead of returning to the Ferry Building, make your return voyage to Fisherman's Wharf. This is a particularly good idea if you'd like to have dinner at the Wharf. A good schedule might be to leave the Ferry Building at 5:15 P.M., arrive in Tiburon at 6:00 P.M., with an 8:00 P.M. departure from Tiburon. You arrive at Fisherman's Wharf at

8:35, in time for a late dinner. (Be sure to check sailing times by calling 546–2815.)

But first, a pre- or post-lunch tour of spectacular **Embarcadero Center,** a multilevel four-building complex, interconnected above street level. Buildings 1, 2, and 3—the ones you want to see—are accessible. You cannot, however, go from 1 to 2 and 3 without returning to street level. What this means is that you enter Embarcadero 3, ascend to the upper podium level, and roll over to Embarcadero 2. You descend to street level from an elevator in building 2. Then at street level you roll from building 2 to Embarcadero 1.

Begin with a visit to 3 Embarcadero Center at Sacramento Street between Davis and Drumm streets. You'll find the elevator near the escalator and the gigantic fabric sculpture entitled "Yellow Legs." When you dial the guard, he sends the elevator down to you. Get off at the second level to see the **Levi Strauss Historical Room,** where is traced the evolution of blue jeans. Then continue your tour of Embarcadero 3 by going via elevator to the top podium level. This level connects with 2 Embarcadero. Explore the shops and, when you're ready to move on, look for the Allrich Gallery, which is near a second elevator. Descend by elevator to the street level and roll west along Sacramento Street to Embarcadero 1, between Battery and Front streets. The elevator that will take you to this podium level is located opposite McGrath Jewelers.

Over $2 million was committed to beautifying the Center. The result is a wealth of original tapestries, paintings, and sculptures. The most recent commission to be completed is the magnificent five-story "Sky Tree" sculpture, a metal mobile that catches sunlight, reflects it, and then colors it with lights. Don't miss the impressive Hemisphere Fountain in Alcoa Plaza to the north. The fountain, made up of 115 stems each producing an umbrella of water, forms a dome of water.

For lunch choose between such accessible restaurants as the **Holding Company Restaurant** or **Salmagundi Restaurant** in building 2 or the **Crisis Hopkins Restaurant** in building 3. There are other possibilities among the street-level restaurant offerings.

Head back in the direction of the Metro subway station, and follow the paved path that runs along the north side of the Hyatt

Regency Hotel to the **Justin Herman Plaza.** Here you'll see the controversial Vaillancourt Fountain. The massive water sculpture, a 710-ton labyrinth of intertwined tentacles that spout 30,000 gallons of water per minute, has been called everything from the ultimate in modern design to "Stonehenge unhinged with plumbing troubles."

Street vendors gather in the plaza each noontime to sell their artwork: macrame, appliques, graphics, feather puppets, and stained glass mirrors. You'll even see some artists working: sketching, tying macrame, working leather. Should you feel like a snack at this point, try the German sausages and sauerkraut vended from the cafe on wheels.

The historic **Ferry Building** across the street from the plaza now houses the World Trade Center. You can tour the building using the steep ramp, as Ironsides did in one of his TV episodes, to see the leftover mosaics and murals from the days when the building was terminus for the Southern Pacific Railroad. Ferry boats carried passengers from the Oakland train station to San Francisco. If you're interested in geology, don't miss the **Mines and Geology Museum** on the second floor, with thousands of minerals, rock and ore specimens. The minerals are arranged according to their chemical content, in one of the largest and most beautiful exhibits in California.

One of the blue and white cruisers may be docked at **Pier 1** just north of the Ferry Building, waiting to carry you to Tiburon. Since ferries bound for Sausalito and Larkspur also leave from this pier, be sure you're piped aboard the right vessel.

Underway, you'll come about in the shadow of the San Francisco–Oakland Bay Bridge, skirt the towering hulls of the liners loading along the Embarcadero, then strike a course past Alcatraz, once an infamous prison island. Cruising on, you'll view the Golden Gate Bridge. Its graceful span and its superb setting have made most people shake their heads in agreement with the consensus that it is "the most beautiful bridge in the world." Passing Sausalito, with its rustic houses cascading down steep slopes, you'll turn east onto Raccoon Strait and the port of **Tiburon.**

You'll want to ramble down Main Street to see the imaginative shops and stop at a waterfront cafe. Among the accessible favorites is **Sam's,** a down-home easy-going spot where you'll find your place in the sun while sipping their famed gin fizzes. Another good bet is **Sabella's Restaurant,** with its lovely outdoor deck.

When your ship comes in to carry you back to San Francisco, settle comfortably on deck for the nighttime view of the skyline. See how many of the buildings you can recognize.

When you dock at the **Wharf,** you'll be within feet of the shops and restaurants. Should food be on your mind, San Francisco natives want to keep it quiet, but **Scoma's** is the place to go. It's a little off the beaten track in an alley off Jefferson Street. Since they don't take reservations, you'll have to take your chances. An alternate is a lovely restaurant nearby, **Castagnola's,** famed for its fresh salmon, sea bass, petrale, and halibut.

After dinner, should your eyes still be open, cross the street for a look inside the magic shop next to the **World of the Unexplained.** The young people behind the counters are all aspiring magicians who will happily demonstrate tricks using Chinese rings, hot rods, or sponge balls. Having seen these mysteries, if anyone asks you about San Francisco you can call it a city of magic and know you are not falling into the usual cliche.

## TOUR 2

WHAT YOU'LL DO

- Lunch at the Garden Court, Sheraton Palace Hotel.
* - Attend a Thursday afternoon performance of the San Francisco Symphony Orchestra.
* - Visit the San Francisco Museum of Modern Art (closed Mondays).
- Tour Japan Center and dine at the East-West Dining Room, Miyako Hotel.

HOW YOU'LL DO IT

- Push to Embarcadero or Civic Center BART station.
- Push from Montgomery Street BART station one block to Sheraton Palace Hotel, 639 Market Street. Use New Mont-

* Indicates restriction in time of visit.
† All sites listed under "Restrooms" offer accessible facilities with wide stall doors and grab bars unless otherwise indicated.

gomery Street entrance (two steps, but doorman pleased to assist).

- Cab from Hotel to Opera House, Van Ness Avenue at Civic Center.
- Push a half block to Museum of Modern Art, Van Ness Avenue.
- Cab from Museum to Japan Center, enter East Building facing Miyako Hotel parking lot on Post Street.
- Cab from Center to your hotel.

### THINGS TO KNOW

- Lunch served in the Garden Court from 11:30 A.M. to 2:30 P.M., Monday–Friday. Reservations advised.
* - San Francisco Symphony Orchestra season runs December–May, with Thursday afternoon concerts at 2:00 P.M. Tickets often available on day of performance, but best to reserve and mention you are in a wheelchair.
* - Museum of Modern Art open Tuesday–Friday 10:00 A.M–10:00 P.M., Saturday–Sunday 10:00 A.M.–5:00 P.M. Admission free. Cafe open 10:00 A.M.–4:00 P.M.

### RESTROOMS †

- Civic Center BART station
- Civic Center, across from Opera House (accessible, but stalls only 25 inches. Enter via vehicle ramp to side of Grove Street.)
- Opera House (restrooms accessible, but stalls less than 25 inches)

Back in 1875, when Nevada silver mine money poured into San Francisco and the bonanza kings and queens ate off solid gold plates, the world's grandest hotel, the opulent **Palace Hotel,** opened its richly carved doors. Today its courtyard, once used as the hotel's carriage entrance, is preserved as a historical monument. Happily it's a monument you can savor in more ways than one.

You should make reservations in advance for lunch at the Palace. Enter by the main entrance, which is on New Montgomery. An affable doorman will assist you up the two steps into the posh red-carpeted lobby. Beyond mirrored doors, under a five-story-high canopy of glass, is the famed **Garden Court.** One hopes that the sun will be shining, brightening the room of polished, gold-touched walls, chandeliers, and marble columns that date back to 1875. Potted palms, fresh flowers, shining crystal, and impeccable table linens complete the sumptuous mood.

Unfortunately the food does not match the superb ambience. You can, however, count on the Palace Court Salad, a medley of artichoke hearts, crab or shrimp, and Louis dressing. Or try the most famous of the menu offerings, the Green Goddess Salad, invented here in 1915. The lettuce topped with shrimp or crab is still dressed in the memorable blend of mayonnaise, anchovy, and tarragon created as a tribute to stage actor George Arliss.

Before continuing on from the hotel, stop to look into the Pied Piper Bar to see its huge, original Maxwell Parrish painting.

As you drive from the hotel to the Opera House you'll pass through the city's Civic Center, a group of buildings fringed by trees, fountains, and plazas. Across the street from the impressive City Hall reign twin buildings—the **Opera House** and the War Memorial Veteran's Building. The Opera House, built in the European tradition, opened in 1932 and has since been the cultural hub of the city. The San Francisco Symphony Orchestra, based here from December to May, shares the spacious house with the equally famed San Francisco Opera Company and the award-winning San Francisco Ballet. If you're lucky you may be able to attend a concert in which the new conductor, Edo de Waart, introduces the work of a contemporary American composer or leads the orchestra in its premiere performance of some other masterwork.

After the last bow, continue your tour by rolling a half block to the War Memorial Veterans Building. Visit the **San Francisco Museum of Art** by riding the elevator to the fourth floor. The museum, famous as a West Coast pioneer in abstract art, remains the nucleus of modern art in the San Francisco Bay area. See the latest showing of works by local painters, sculptors, and printmakers, plus the contemporary graphics and photographs exhibited on the third floor. The museum also houses a permanent collection distinguished by works of Matisse, Klee, Alexander Calder, Jackson Pollock, and Clyfford Still. As you leave, don't miss the museum shop on the first floor.

As you continue by cab to the Japan Center you'll climb Cathedral Hill, dominated by the stunning **St. Mary's Cathedral.** The startling contours of the shining white exterior have inspired such descriptions as "washing machine agitator" or "the Taj taking off." The Cathedral is accessible, if you'd like to stop for a look at the radiant stained glass windows that extend 139 feet down the four sides to shape a multicolored cruciform.

Down the hill and you're at the **Japan Center,** with its Ginza-like array of restaurants, teahouses, shops, and theaters. The Center was designed by Minoru Yamasaki, who also designed the World Trade Center and the Century Plaza Hotel in Los Angeles. The highlights here are Peace Plaza and the Peace Pagoda, landscaped with Japanese gardens and reflecting pools. A copper-roofed walkway connects this hub with the two buildings filled with Japanese shops, showrooms, bookstores, art galleries, and restaurants.

You can wheel around the three-block center looking into the shops carrying the most extensive collection of Japanese goods outside the Orient—everything from live carp and dwarfed bonsai trees to woodcut prints and oysters with pearls inside. Begin by entering the East Building that opens onto the Miyako Hotel parking lot. Explore the street level second floor area of this building and then take an elevator down to the garden level. From the garden level you can exit via a steep slope to the garden and then continue on to the Kintetsu Building with its indoor bridge spanning Webster Street. The bridge, inspired by Florence's Ponte Vecchio, shelters a Japanese doll-making school and art galleries, including one that exhibits selected works from the Avery Brundage Collection of Asian Art.

As you explore you might like to see the academy that teaches classes in Japanese flower arranging, brush painting, the tea ceremony, batik, calligraphy, and the game of Go.

For dinner you can choose from a number of accessible restaurants including the **Miyako Hotel's East-West Dining Room.** The lovely room offers an overview of a lovely sunken garden plus authentic Japanese cuisine served by kimono-clad waitresses.

## TOUR 3

WHAT YOU'LL DO

- View the city from Twin Peaks.
- Visit Golden Gate Park, with a stop at the Conservatory, M. H. deYoung Memorial Museum, the Japanese Tea Garden, California Academy of Sciences, and the Aquarium.
- Drive along the Pacific Ocean portion of the 49-Mile Scenic Drive, continuing over Golden Gate Bridge to Sausalito.
- Dine overlooking the bay at the Valhalla Inn.
- Take an after-dinner ramble along the waterfront.

HOW YOU'LL DO IT

- Drive from your hotel to Golden Gate Park.
- Push around Park concourse, visiting the deYoung Museum, California Academy of Sciences, and the Japanese Tea Garden.
- Drive from concourse to park's Conservatory of Flowers— use side entrance to left off Kennedy Drive.
- Drive along the Great Highway, Pt. Lobos Avenue and Lincoln Boulevard, over the Golden Gate Bridge to Sausalito, taking Alexander Avenue exit.
- Drive into downtown Sausalito and then to the Valhalla Inn, 201 Bridgeway.
- Drive from the restaurant to your hotel.

THINGS TO KNOW

- Good idea to bring a picnic for lunch.
- Park buildings open 10:00 A.M.–5:00 P.M. daily. DeYoung Museum 75¢/25¢. Academy of Sciences 50¢/25¢. Conservatory free. Japanese Tea Garden free.
- Lunch served in deYoung Museum restaurant.
- Valhalla Inn requires dinner reservations.

$___/$___ indicates adult/child admission fees.
† All sites listed under "Restrooms" offer accessible facilities with wide stall doors and grab bars unless otherwise indicated.

RESTROOMS †

- California Academy of Sciences.
- DeYoung Museum, Conservatory of Flowers (accessible restrooms but stalls less than 25 inches wide)

No visit to San Francisco would be complete without a view from Twin Peaks, a visit to Golden Gate Park, and a drive along the Pacific Coast. All three of these attractions are included in the 49-Mile Scenic Drive that links the city's most important scenic and historic points. A good map of this famous drive is the free "San Francisco Visitors Map" available by request from the Visitors Bureau. Although the drive can be made in half a day, that doesn't include much time in Golden Gate Park. So instead of doing the whole drive, perhaps you'll want to hit the most spectacular portions and give yourself plenty of time to tour the park and see its several must-see attractions. By doing this you'll cover new ground, see the highlights of the 49-Mile Scenic Drive, have time at Golden Gate Park—and you'll only have to rent a car for one day.

Although the views are spectacular on this full-day tour, the accessible restaurants where you can have lunch are limited. You can lunch at the deYoung Museum restaurant, but more appropriate, perhaps, is a picnic lunch. See if your hotel can pack one.

Begin by driving out Market Street to 14th Street, which curves into Roosevelt Way and Twin Peaks Boulevard. From the 900-foot north or south summits of **Twin Peaks,** you'll see the city spread at your feet. Market Street was surveyed from between the two peaks to run in a straight line to the Ferry Building.

From Twin Peaks continue along Twin Peaks Boulevard to Woodside Avenue, Laguna Honda Boulevard and Parnassus Avenue to Stanyan Street and the Panhandle entrance to **Golden Gate Park.** The Panhandle, once a carriage promenade, is lined by some of the city's oldest trees.

By staying to the right on Kennedy Drive, you'll come to the glass **Conservatory of Flowers.** The enchanting structure, a copy of the Royal Conservatories in London's Kew Gardens, was built for a private estate and later purchased by San Francisco citizens for their park. Use the side entrance to see the interior with its huge pool filled with water lilies, the hybrid orchid exhibit, and beautifully arranged seasonal blooms.

The hub of the park is a short distance from the Conservatory. To reach it, pass the Rhododendron Dell and take the road that leads south at 9th Avenue. Clustered around a music concourse with a bandshell and neat rows of plane trees are the Japanese Tea Garden, deYoung Museum, and the Academy of Sciences.

Beyond a gate made of hundreds of hand-carved pieces of hinoki wood lies the serene **Japanese Tea Garden** that could have been transplanted from Kyoto. In a sense it was when in 1894 an Oriental art importer brought in workmen and materials directly from Japan to create this four-acre glen. Lichened rockeries, stone lanterns, muted blue and gold torii portals, a bronze Buddha, an arched moon bridge, and a five-tiered pagoda are part of the result. So are the decorative flora collected from throughout the Orient: dwarf maples, azaleas and conifers, evergreen bamboo, flowering cherry, peach, plum, and quince trees. About half of the garden can be seen by a wheeler on his or her own. Another fourth is accessible but requires assistance. With assistance you can also visit the thatched Japanese tea house, where kimono-clad girls serve specially blended tea and cookies. The garden can also be appreciated from the floor-to-ceiling windows in the **Asian Art Museum** that overlook it.

The Asian Art Museum, in a wing of the **deYoung Memorial Museum,** houses what may be the greatest collection of Oriental art in the Western world. The collection spans sixty centuries. The Museum is most noteworthy for its fine period rooms, including ones from a French chateau, an Italian alpine chalet, and an Elizabethan oak-paneled hall.

In 1977 the deYoung opened its new wing exhibiting American art, which includes a parlor from an 1805-vintage Massachusetts home. Of special interest is the newest gallery showing the arts of Africa, Oceania, and the Americas.

If your visit to the park precedes the deYoung Museum's planned completion of a ramp at the front entrance, go around the back of the Museum to the loading dock area, where the guard on duty will admit you through the level rear entrance.

The **California Academy of Sciences,** across from the museum,

houses within its walls a major aquarium, planetarium, and numerous halls of science. If nothing else, see the unique Fish Round-
about, a doughnut-shaped tank that you can roll up into. This unusual structure, since it has no middle portion as conventional circular tanks do, causes the fish to swim around rather than across
the tank. This means you get a better look at the fish, and probably
the fish are happier since they believe they are swimming in a
linear stream and not simply around in circles.

After a picnic lunch beside the Academy's beautiful outdoor
fountain or in the deYoung Museum, continue your tour of Golden
Gate Park by driving its length and breadth. As you drive through
miles of glens, meadows, and gardens, you'll find it difficult to
believe that this sylvan scene was once one big sand dune. For
years after the city purchased the land in 1868, the park remained
a hopeless wasteland where the sand buried all greenery. Only
through the determination of William Hammond Hall, a devoted
horticulturist who also happened to be park superintendent, did the
three-mile-long strip of desolation begin to support the plants and
trees he planted—and replanted. Today you see many of the old
trees he planted, and some of the 5,000 different kinds of plants
that carpet the land go back to his time.

As you tour this man-made wonder, look for the buffalo pad-
dock, Stow Lake, Spreckels Lake, and the two great stone wind-
mills. If time permits, stop at the accessible **Strybing Arboretum
and Botanical Garden,** with its hard-surfaced paths leading through
sixty acres of more than 6000 species of plants.

When you're ready to leave, take South Drive to 47th Street and
follow Fulton Street toward the ocean. **The Great Highway** sweeps
along the oceanfront for three miles, affording open-ended views of
the crashing waves. You can stop at several points along the highway to look out to sea, perhaps focusing on the hang gliders
near Fort Funston to the south. On clear days Farallon Islands,
twenty-seven miles offshore, are visible. Almost any day you can
spot sea lions splashing around the nearby northwestern cliffs, or
surfers at Kelly's Cove.

As you continue to follow the 49-Mile-Drive, you'll turn into
Lincoln Park with its magnificent **Palace of the Legion of Honor,** a
replica of its Paris namesake. From the plateau fronting the Pal-

ace, you'll see one of the most stunning views of the Golden Gate Bridge, probably your first view from its western side. Lincoln Drive curls along the coast, passing more points for enjoying views of the bridge with waves dashing at its feet. Drive off the side roads that lead to Phelan or Baker Beach for even more views of the bridge, the sea, and the green hills of Marin.

Lincoln Drive hooks up with Highway 101, which will carry you across the bridge to Sausalito.

Near the **Golden Gate Bridge** toll plaza you can, if you're hearty and adventurous, park and ask a guard to unlock the gate to the pedestrian walkway that crosses the bridge. By rolling along even a few feet you'll get a grand view and an invigorating breath of fresh air. Even on a day that's calm everywhere else in this city, the wind is alive and kicking on the Golden Gate Bridge.

Once a fishing village, **Sausalito** is now the choice of many writers and artists. Rustic houses hang on the steep slopes and seem about to cascade into the bay.

Before stopping at the Valhalla Inn, drive down Bridgeway Drive into the town center with its arty shops, ferry boat store, and charming town plaza.

As you turn back up Bridgeway you'll follow a seaside board-walk that leads directly to the **Valhalla Inn.** The restaurant is owned by Sally Stanford, a former madam. When Sally went "legit," she opened the Valhalla and, amazingly enough, became mayor in 1975. Her bayside restaurant is fascinating, filled with a wild assortment of Victorian antiques and turn-of-the-century bric-a-brac.

After dinner and a ramble along the boardwalk, continue back to San Francisco, with a stop at Vista Point on the Marin side of the bridge for a look at the skyline. This will be a good time to review what you've seen and to decide what you will see again— and again—when you come back for your heart!

## Other Accessible Attractions

Brooks Hall, Larkin & McAllister streets (use ramp from second-floor Civic Center garage)
Cable Car Museum, 1201 Mason Street

California Palace of Legion of Honor, Lincoln Park (three steps at entrance; 1st-floor exhibits only)

Candlestick Park, home of the 49ers and Giants (steep ramp)

Civic Auditorium, Grove Street at Civic Center

Coit Tower, Telegraph Hill (terrace only)

Curran Theater, 445 Geary Street (two steps at entrance)

Geary Theater, 415 Geary Street (two steps at entrance)

Harbor Tours, pier 43½ at Fisherman's Wharf

Marina Green & Yacht Harbor, Marina Boulevard at Baker Street

Marine's Memorial, 609 Sutter Street

Masonic Auditorium, 1111 California Street

North Point Shopping Center, Bay and Stockton Street (enter from parking lot)

Orpheum Theater, 1192 Market Street

Stern Grove, 19th Avenue and Sloat Boulevard (access via long steep descent)

Wells Fargo Museum, 420 Montgomery Street (enter thru California Street door)

Winterland, Post and Steiner (level access)

Zoological Gardens, Zoo Road and Skyline Boulevard (enter via Skyline Boulevard)

INTRODUCING
*Rollin' On* adviser, wheeler John Edmonds

*Title:* Chairman, Board of Control, San Francisco Muni (Transportation) Handicapped & Elderly Study

*Hometown:* San Francisco

*Favorite tourist site:* The *Balclutha* sailing ship

*Hidden corner:* Stow Lake, Golden Gate Park

*Rendezvous:* Iron Horse in Maiden Lane

*Offbeat restaurant:* Tommy's Joynt

*Place for music:* American Music Hall

*View:* from Twin Peaks

*Natural wonder:* San Francisco Bay as seen from the middle of the Golden Gate Bridge

*Museum:* San Francisco Museum of Modern Art

*Ramble:* the flat 2–3 mile stretch that skirts the Bay along The Embarcadero. Begin at the Ferry Building and stop for a beer at Pier 23. Route ends at Fisherman's Wharf

*Non-tourist destination:* Mission Street between 16th and 29th streets (get there via BART)

*Offbeat experience:* the Dicken's Christmas Faire held at the Cow Palace in December

*Traditional restaurant:* Scoma's or Schroeder's Cafe

*Low-cost restaurant:* Stone Soup or Salmagundi's

*Ice cream shop:* Swenson's

*Reading suggestion: Mirror of the Dream, Illustrated History of San Francisco* by Roger Olmstead & Tom Watkins

*Place to get a wheelchair repaired:* Abbey Rents

*Tip on having a great time in San Francisco:* Plan to eat and drink a lot and don't try to do too much. Stop and observe. The natives are friendly. Ask strangers where they're from and you'll probably find someone who just moved to San Francisco from your hometown!

# 12

# Washington, D.C.

Seeing Washington, D.C., for the first time is like meeting an old friend on the street after many years. In real life this old friend of a city not only looks familiar but stirs forgotten feelings. Pictures of her marble monuments, her bronze statues, her sweeping paths of greenery are etched in the mind, as are the patriotism and pride we felt as youngsters on first hearing the stories of our country's famous leaders.

Who does not know that compassionate face of the seated Lincoln looking beyond his marble Parthenon to the Reflecting Pool? Who has not memorized the silhouette of the Washington Monument and of the Capitol on its hilltop perch? Who has not come to know as intimately as his own home the stately proportions of the White House with its lighted portico?

The traveler to our nation's capital feels that he has come home and, in actuality, he has. For as a citizen—and as a tax payer—the monuments, the government buildings, the federal parks, the museums, art galleries, and even a zoo belong to him. And because they do, best of all, they're free.

Few cities offer more to see and do at no cost than does this federal city. One could spend months or years exploring the wealth inside its repositories. More time could be spent discovering its dozens of graceful city squares with flowers and shady trees, the rolling greensward that is the Mall, the leafy banks of the Potomac River.

And the history symbolized in its monuments, the America of

yesterday preserved in its museums, and its abundance of parks and vistas are only part of the whole. Washington, D.C. is also an exciting twentieth-century city, an important center where news of worldwide importance is made every day. The mighty from throughout the world are attracted to this capital, as are many who strive for change through demonstrations or through meetings with legislators.

The tourist becomes part of the news simply because he is for a time present. He stops to talk with a demonstrator in front of the White House, glimpses a newsmaker entering the Executive Office Building, dines a table away from a senator or congressman, or thinks he recognizes the face behind the window of the black limousine with diplomatic license plates.

At night lights shine. The Kennedy Center for the Performing Arts vies with New York's Lincoln Center and Broadway for the quality and diversity of its entertainment. Four theaters present concerts, plays, opera, ballet and motion pictures. In addition, little theater groups offer a broad variety of fare, including the three theaters that make up the much-lauded Arena Stage repertory company. Dinner theaters abound in the suburbs. In the summer Wolf Trap Farm Park, the Margaret Merriweather Post Pavilion, and the Carter Barron Amphitheater stage musical events. Throughout the year concerts—many free of charge—are presented at the Library of Congress, the Smithsonian, the National Gallery of Art, the Renwick Gallery, Constitution Hall, and Lisner Auditorium. Jazz and folk nightclubs and rock and soul clubs in the downtown and Georgetown area supplement the entertainment spectrum.

With this variety of entertainment and sightseeing attractions by day, Washington, D.C., offers something for everyone.

For the wheelchair traveler the city affords unusual accessibility, thanks to the opening in 1977 of twenty-one miles of Metro subway track with twenty-nine stations. Metro opens the capital to the handicapped person, making it possible for him or her to see almost every major tourist sight. This accessibility, combined with the relatively good access to government buildings and the flatness of the city, make it one of the best destinations for the wheelchair traveler.

## Planning Your Trip

Any Washingtonian will tell you that the time to visit the capital is in the spring or fall. Summer is too hot, winter too cold; fall and spring are just right. But in the spring crowds are at their peak and seeing the sights and getting around take patience. Fall actually is more ideal, for during this season the weather is at its most predictable best (little rain), and the trees turning flamboyant red, yellow, and orange color the city. Days are crisp, not cold but not hot either. Crowds are fewer, especially after Labor Day.

In planning your trip any time of year, you'll want to write to your senator or congressman requesting a bid for the VIP tour of the White House. Allow at least one month from his receipt of your letter before you want to take the tour. When you're writing, ask also for a ticket to the House or Senate so that when you visit the Capitol you'll be able to drop in on a session.

You might also consider writing to the Smithsonian Institution requesting a Resident Associate membership. For $18 you'll receive the beautiful *Smithsonian* magazine, a newsletter listing lectures, tours, and special events, and a card entitling you to a 10 percent discount on souvenirs, books, art reproductions, toys, and many other items available in the many Smithsonian gifts shops.

Seeing the diplomatic reception rooms of the Department of State has to be one of the least known thrills of a visit to Washington. To see a remarkable collection of antiques in a superb setting, write one month ahead to the Tour Department, Department of State, 2200 C Street, N.W., Washington, D.C. 20037. Give the day you wish to come and whether you will join the 9:30, 10:30 A.M. or 3:30 P.M. tour. (See Tour 6 itinerary for time suggestion.)

To receive a listing of future performances at the Kennedy Center, write to the Friends of the Kennedy Center, Kennedy Center for Performing Arts, Washington, D.C. 20566. You can order tickets before you arrive, but you may instead want to take advantage of the 50 percent discount on most performances offered to handicapped visitors who come to the Friends of the Kennedy Center desk and request the coupon, which can be applied to the cost of tickets.

For information and maps of the city write to the Washington

Area Convention and Visitors Bureau, 1129 20th Street N.W., Suite 200, Washington, D.C. 20036. *Access Washington* is available from the Information Center for Handicapped Individuals, 1413 K Street N.W., Twelfth Floor, Washington, D.C. 20005.

Finally, when packing include a raincoat, an extra sweater, and a warm scarf or hat. Washington weather is unpredictable and even a sunny warm day can turn into a cold one with no warning. More than in almost any other city it will pay to be prepared with a variety of clothing you can shed or add to as the day or evening gets warmer or cooler.

### How to Get There

Washington, D.C., is served by Greyhound, Trailways, Amtrak, and major airlines.

Greyhound has a downtown station at 12th Street and New York Avenue N.W., about four blocks from the White House. Entrances are level and a restroom is accessible next to the baggage pickup area. Taxis are usually outside the main door. Although it might be tempting to push yourself to a downtown hotel or to the Metro subway station at 14th and I streets, don't. This area of town, although not unusually dangerous, is seedy.

Union Station, the terminus for Amtrak train service, is located at the foot of the Capitol, about a mile from the White House. At Union Station you'll find accessible restrooms and available taxicabs.

Three airports serve the District, two of them about twenty-seven miles from downtown: Dulles International Airport in Virginia and Baltimore-Washington International Airport; the third, Washington National Airport in Virginia, is three miles from downtown Washington. All offer accessible restrooms. Because of the distance involved when arriving at the Dulles or Baltimore-Washington airports, it's a good idea to book a flight arriving at National Airport even though that might mean changing planes at some point en route. That way you'll save the $20 cab fare charges for the Dulles or Baltimore-Washington airports to D.C. run and pay instead only about $4 for the National Airport to D.C. ride.

If you are coming to Washington by car, be sure to avoid the weekday rush hour traffic from 7:00 to 9:00 A.M. and 4:00 to 6:00 P.M. Also, since interstate freeways in and around the city seem constantly to be in various transition stages, be sure you have a recent state highway map. A good one is issued periodically by the District of Columbia Department of Transportation, but they're not mailed out, so ask a friend to pick one up for you at 415 12th Street, N.W.

### Getting Around Washington

Traffic congestion and shortages of parking spaces make car travel in the District a frustrating experience. Once in town, the best idea may be to park your car and use the Metro subway and taxicabs.

After fifty years of talk, millions of man-hours of toil, and the expenditure of $5 billion, you'd expect it to be pretty good. But Washington's Metro subway is more than good, it's an entirely new transportation experience. It's fun.

The stations themselves are beautiful, most with coffered ceilings that remind you of the Pantheon dome. The quality of design is only matched by the humanistic character of the whole operation. A great deal of thought went into making both the trains and the stations quiet, climate-controlled, safe, and comfortable.

After you've taken your first ride you may agree that experiencing the Metro subway alone is worth a trip to the capital. Of course, the entire system is totally accessible. One entrance at each subway stop offers elevator access to the underground network. At some you simply push the button and the elevator conveys you to the lobby, where you purchase your farecard. At others you push the "talk" button and speak with the station attendant before descending directly to the station platform.

You can write ahead for the *All About Metro* brochure and the flyer telling how handicapped persons and senior citizens can take advantage of the Metro's reduced fare program. Address your information request to the Washington Metropolitan Area Transit Authority, 600 5th Street N.W., Washington, D.C. 20001

## Metro Station Handicapped Elevator Entrances

### Red Line Stations

| | |
|---|---|
| Rhode Island Avenue | *Rhode Island Ave. & 8th St., N.E.* |
| Union Station-Visitor Center | *Mass. Ave & 1st St., N.E.* |
| Judiciary Square | *F St. Between 4th and 5th Sts., N.W.* |
| Gallery Place | *\*SE corner of 7th & G Sts., N.W.* |
| Metro Center | *NE corner of 12th & G Sts., N.W.* |
| Farragut North | *SE corner of Conn. Ave. & K St., N.W.* |
| Dupont Circle | *SW corner of Conn. Ave. & Q St., N.W.* |

### Blue Line Stations

| | |
|---|---|
| National Airport | *Opposite the North Terminal* |
| Crystal City | *North of 18th St., East of Clark St.* |
| Pentagon City | *East side of Hayes St. between Army-Navy and 15th St.* |
| Pentagon | *East end of bus island* |
| Arlington Cemetery | *North side of Memorial Drive, west of Jeff Davis Hwy.* |
| Rosslyn | *East side of N. Moore between 19th & Wilson* |
| Foggy Bottom | *North side of Eye between 23rd & 24th Sts., N.W.* |
| Farragut West | *NW corner of 18th & Eye Sts., N.W.* |
| McPherson Square | *SW corner of 14th & Eye Sts., N.W.* |
| Metro Center (Transfer Station) | *East side of 12th St., north of G St., N.W.* |

| | |
|---|---|
| Federal Triangle | *West side of 12th St. between Penn. & Constitution Aves., N.W.* |
| Smithsonian | *North of Independence Ave., west of 12th St., S.W.* |
| L'Enfant Plaza | *7th St. and C St., S.W.* |
| Federal Center, S.W. | *SW corner of D & 3rd Sts., S.W.* |
| Capitol South | *West of 1st St., between C & D Sts., S.W.* |
| Eastern Market | *East of 7th St. and South of Penn. Ave., S.E.* |
| Potomac Avenue | *East side of 14th St., S.E., between Potomac Ave. & G St., S.E.* |
| Stadium/Armory | *19th & C Sts., S.E.* |

The Metro subway operates on weekdays only from 6:30 A.M. to 8:00 P.M. All itineraries in this chapter that suggest the use of the Metro subway are planned for non-rush hour times: 9:30 A.M. to 3:30 P.M. and 6:00 to 8:00 P.M. At non-rush hour times the fare is 40¢, but cash cannot be used. Instead one purchases a fare card by depositing coins or bills in the machines at each station. You'll find it a time saver if you purchase a $4 ticket allowing you to ride the subway ten times while you're in Washington, rather than a series of 40¢ tickets each time you ride.

The Metro subway network is made up of two different lines, the Red Line, linking stations within the District, and the Blue Line, linking additional District stations and portions of Virginia. You must, of course, know whether it is the Blue or Red Line you'll be riding and if it will be necessary to transfer.

In planning your itinerary, note the color of the line serving your destination. If the station where you board is served by the same color line, that's it. But if your destination is on the Blue Line, you'll have to transfer at Metro Center—the only place you can transfer—which is different from other stations in that it has a double ceiling instead of the standard single one.

Once you're straight about Blue and Red lines, your only other consideration will be getting yourself on a train going the right direction. How do you know what the right direction is? You must know that trains are marked with the name of the last station on either end of the Red or Blue Line. So all you do is locate your boarding station and your destination on the map and note the name of the last station that lies in the direction opposite to where you are boarding. Thus, if you board the Metro subway at Farragut West and are going to Rosslyn, you'll see on the map that National Airport is the final station in your chosen direction and you board the train marked "National Airport." Of course, everyone asks questions of everyone else so you may find yourself answering a few questions if you look less than confused. If you're not sure, ask other passengers or the Metro personnel stationed throughout the subway.

Taxicabs, used extensively in the suggested Washington itineraries here, are plentiful and fares are relatively low. Taxicabs in the District compute fares on the zone system rather than the usual metered mileage gauge, which explains why you'll on occasion get a long ride for your money. Playing the zone game is an art usually reserved for long-term Washingtonians. However, by looking at the map posted on back of the driver's seat you'll get a clue on how you could start playing.

As a one-time swampland (before being filled in as the site of our nation's capital), Washington, D.C., is almost entirely flat, with the exceptions of Capitol Hill and parts of Georgetown. For the wheelchair traveler this means care-free pushing. To add to the relative ease of getting around, the District also offers a good network of curb cuts. The twenty-block-long Mall, stretching between the U.S. Capitol and the Lincoln Memorial, is totally ramped between 3rd and 14th streets, and almost completely cut the rest of the way. In other parts of the city, as old curbs are repaired, new ramps are cut. The number is constantly increasing, with the result that you can almost always find a cut where you need it.

Building ramps, too, are more plentiful in Washington than they are in many other cities, since all new federal buildings must comply with the 1968 law that requires accessible entries to public buildings. During the Bicentennial, many of the older federal buildings—including the museums on the Mall—set up ramps; but sometimes the doors beyond these ramps are locked so the wheelchair traveler must ask (or telephone ahead) for assistance in having the door opened.

## Where to Stay

Because the Metro subway is such an ideal means for the wheelchair traveler to get around Washington, its seems logical to stay at a hotel near one of its stations. Happily, there are a number of accessible hotels within a block or two of the subway: the Mayflower Hotel, one block from the Farragut North station; the Hyatt Regency Hotel, three easy blocks from the Union Station subway stop; the Marriott–Crystal City, next to the Crystal City Metro station.

The **Mayflower Hotel,** 1127 Connecticut Avenue N.W., is hard to beat for comfort and gracious European style. There's a touch of elegance and a sense of history in this venerable institution that has catered to presidents and kings. Included among the extensive facilities is one of the city's highest rated restaurants, The Carvery, a lovely room of sixteenth-century Spanish motif famous for its steaks and prime ribs. The hotel offers all the amenities plus special rooms for wheelchair guests.

The **Hyatt Regency Hotel** at 400 New Jersey Avenue N.W. is a modified version of the chain's famed hotels in San Francisco and Atlanta. Guest rooms line balconies that overlook an atrium lobby highlighted by a flower-filled sidewalk cafe. Linking the lobby with the rooftop view restaurant is a glass elevator. A ramped entrance right next to the main entrance gives wheelchair travelers access to the elevator that descends to the lobby or ascends to guest rooms and the rooftop restaurant.

The hotel features seven specially designed rooms for disabled visitors. These have lowered light switches, hand-held shower spigots, and direct closet access. Curb ramps on New Jersey Avenue and D and North Capitol streets make access to the Metro subway at Union Station feasible.

The **Marriott–Crystal City,** 1999 Jefferson Davis Highway, Arlington, Virginia, is a block and a half and several curb cuts away from the Crystal City Metro subway station. From the subway elevator entrance the wheeler can roll a few yards to the buildings that give elevator access to the Crystal City Underground, a complex of forty-five shops and restaurants. The Marriott Hotel offers such amenities as courtesy limousine service from nearby National Airport, a restaurant overlooking the Plaza, a pool, and patio. Special weekend and family rates are available.

For visitors with their own transportation, there's the **Sheraton Park Hotel** at 2660 Woodley Road N.W. This hotel put $75,000 into creating a model barrier-free environment for the 1977 White House Conference on Handicapped Individuals. Unfortunately the hotel is situated several miles from the sightseeing heart of the District and there is no wheelchair-accessible means of transportation available except taxicab or one's own rented car.

Among the other hotels offering special wheelchair guest rooms are:

> Washington Hilton Hotel, 1919 Connecticut Avenue N.W., Washington, D.C.
>
> Howard Johnson's, 2650 Jefferson Davis Highway, Arlington, Virginia
>
> Howard Johnson's, 5811 Annapolis Road, Cheverly, Maryland
>
> Hyatt Hotel, 1325 Wilson Boulevard, Arlington, Virginia
>
> Marriott Hotel, Key Bridges, Rosslyn, Virginia
>
> Metropolitan Hotel, 1143 New Hampshire Avenue N.W., Washington, D.C.

## What You'll See and Do

With six days you'll really see Washington, from Capitol Hill to the Lincoln Memorial, from the Southwest riverfront to the heights of Washington Cathedral. You'll see the major tourist sights and also catch the flavor of this exciting city as you spend a Sunday afternoon on the Mall, tour the elegant State Department reception rooms, and cruise the Potomac River.

Itineraries are suggested based on the special offerings at various sites which are available only on certain days. The use of the Metro has been planned for weekdays and during non-rush hours.

In the evenings you'll enjoy great music and theater, attending a performance at the Kennedy Center, a concert at the National Gallery of Art, a jazz set at Georgetown's famed Blue's Alley.

For dinner you'll choose from great French, Italian, Chinese, American, and seafood restaurants. Among them, these accessible favorites within the District line:

American
    Blackie's, 22nd and M streets N.W. (one step)
    Bassin's, 14th and Pennsylvania Avenue N.W.
    Billy Martin's Carriage House, 1238 Wisconsin Avenue N.W.
    The Foundry, 1050 30th Street N.W.
    The Palm, 1225 19th Street N.W.
    Port o' Georgetown, 1054 31st Street N.W.
    Rumor's, 1900 M Street N.W.
    Scholl's Colonial Cafeteria, 1032 Connecticut Avenue N.W.
        (one step)
    Duke Zeibert's Restaurant, 1722 L Street N.W.

Chinese
    Chin's, 2614 Connecticut Avenue N.W.
    Kowloon, 1105 H Street N.W.
    Moon Palace, 3308 Wisconsin Avenue N.W.
    Yenching, 3524 Connecticut Avenue N.W.

Continental
    Adam's Rib, 2100 Pennsylvania Avenue N.W.
    Bull 'n Bear, 819 15th Street N.W.
    Cafe Burgundy, 5031 Connecticut Avenue N.W.
    Golden Table, 528 23rd Street N.W.
    Hammel's, 416 10th Street N.W.
    Intrigue, 824 New Hampshire Avenue N.W.
    Paul Young's, 1120 Connecticut Avenue N.W.

English
    Piccadilly, 5510 Connecticut Avenue N.W.
    Dubliner Restaurant, 4 F Street N.W.

French
    Cafe de Paris, 3056 M Street N.W. (two steps)
    Jean Pierre, 1835 K Street N.W. (one step)
    La Nicoise Restaurant, 1721 Wisconsin Avenue N.W. (one
        step)

Le Bagatelle, 2000 K Street N.W.
Le Canard, 3288 M Street N.W.
Le Provencal, 1234 20th Street N.W. (first floor only)
L'Escargot, 3309 Connecticut Avenue N.W.
Napoleon's, 2649 Connecticut Avenue N.W.
Sans Souci, 726 17th Street N.W. (upper floor only)
1789, 1226 36th Street N.W. (one step)

German
Old Europe, 2434 Wisconsin Avenue N.W.

Greek
Astor, 1813 M Street N.W.

Indian
Indian Curry House, 2301 Calvert N.W. (outdoor cafe only)
Siddhartha, 1412 New York Avenue N.W. (one step)

Italian
Alfio's La Trattoria, 5100 Wisconsin Avenue N.W.
Anna Maria's, 1737 Connecticut Avenue N.W.
Gusti's, 1837 M Street N.W. (sidewalk cafe)
Metropolitan Hotel, 1143 New Hampshire Avenue N.W.
Roma, 3419 Connecticut Avenue N.W.
Romeo & Juliet, 2020 K Street N.W.
Tiberio, 1915 K Street N.W.

Seafood
Flagship, 900 Water Street S.W.
Hogates, 9th and Main Street S.W.
Market Inn, 200 E Street S.W.
O'Donnell's, 1221 E Street N.W. (one step)
Sea Fair, 2655 Connecticut Avenue N.W. (one step)

Spanish
El Caribe, 1828 Columbia Avenue N.W.

Vegetarian
Golden Temple, 1521 Connecticut Avenue N.W.
Golden Temple Emporium, 1634 Wisconsin Avenue N.W.
    (one step)

Nature's Way, 1015 18th Street N.W.
Yes, 1039 31st Avenue N.W. (one step)

To find out what's going on around town pick up *Capital* or *This Week* in your hotel, buy the Friday edition of the *Washington Post* with its weekend listings, or obtain the current copy of the *Washingtonian Magazine*.

If you have special questions relating to handicapped travel, call the Union Station Handicapped Visitors Center at (202) 523–1603. *Rollin' On* adviser Diane Lattin at the President's Committee for Employment of the Handicapped will also answer your questions; call her at (202) 653–5010.

## TOUR 1

WHAT YOU'LL DO

- Visit the Hirshorn Art Museum for a conducted tour or self-tour, visit museum shop, purchase box lunch.
- Lunch on the Mall.
- Visit to National Air & Space Museum to see film, planetarium, and museum shop, self-tour; get refreshment in cafeteria.
* • Visit National Gallery of Art, take conducted tour or self-tour, visit museum shop, dine in Gallery cafe, attend Sunday evening concert (mid-September through June).

HOW YOU'LL DO IT

- Cab from hotel to Hirshorn Art Museum (accessible entrance at 8th Street and Independence Avenue S.W.).
- Push across driveway from Hirshorn to Mall.
- Push from Mall one block across 7th Street to Air & Space Museum.
- Push two blocks across Mall to National Gallery of Art, Constitution Avenue at 6th Street N.W. Enter on Constitution Avenue.
- Cab from National Gallery of Art to hotel.

* Indicates restriction in time of visit.
† All sites listed under "Restrooms" offer accessible facilities with wide stall doors and grab bars unless otherwise indicated.

THINGS TO KNOW

- Good box lunches available at basement cafe of Hirshorn or from street vendors selling fast foods. Cafe also available at Air & Space Museum.
- Excellent art reproductions available at low cost at National Gallery of Art museum shop.
- Dinner served at National Gallery of Art cafe or cafeteria from 1:00 to 7:00 P.M. on Sunday evenings.
* • Free evening concert at Garden Court of National Gallery of Art by the National Gallery Symphony Orchestra Sundays at 7:00 P.M., mid-September through June.

RESTROOMS †

- Hirshorn, lower level
- National Air & Space Museum, main level
- National Gallery of Art

Your first day in Washington, a Sunday morning with quiet downtown streets and singing church bells.

After finishing your breakfast at the Hotel, bring along your *Washington Post* or *Star* newspaper and call a cab for a ride to the **Hirshorn Art Museum and Sculpture Garden.** Enter at the Independence and 8th Street entrance, which is level, and use the staff elevators for internal touring. But first note the building itself, a modern cylindrical structure surrounding an inner sculpture court. Inside are works by the great names of twentieth-century American art, with a heavy emphasis on sculpture. The installation is chronological with the oldest pieces in the basement and the more recent pieces on the upper floors. If nothing else, the visitor shouldn't miss wheeling around the first and second floor for an overview of the fine sculpture, the impressive fountain in the courtyard, and a view of the outdoor sculpture garden, which is not accessible because of the flight of stairs.

Before leaving take a look at the museum shop in the basement and buy a box lunch to enjoy under a tree on the Mall. For people-watching few places beat the Mall on a Sunday afternoon—there's even a merry-go-round (in operation through early October) packed with children. If you're lucky the Mall also will be the site for an outdoor art fair or a musical performance. After enjoying the Mall and buying an ice cream from a traveling vendor, head across 7th Street to the **National Air and Space Museum.** Enter by using the ramp to the left of the main entrance.

The National Air and Space Museum, opened in 1976, has become a must on every visitor's list. The twenty-six exhibit halls are devoted to such varied air/space subjects as ballooning, World War I aviation, air traffic control, life in the universe, exhibition flying, and flight to the moon. Among the most famous vehicles on display are the Wright brothers' Kitty Hawk *Flyer*; the *Spirit of St. Louis* that took Charles Lindbergh across the Atlantic Ocean; the Bell X-1, the first plane to break the sound barrier in level flight; and the command module "Columbia" that brought back the Apollo II crew and the lunar rock that is also on display.

Putting space and flight into perspective is the spectacular twenty-six-minute movie "To Fly" that's projected on a five-story-high screen, and the planetarium presentation shown at the Albert Einstein Spacearium.

Before leaving the museum, take a look at the unusual museum shop with its model airplanes and kites. Then stop by the cafeteria for a cup of tea and a lovely view of the Capitol and Mall.

When you're ready to leave, push your way across the Mall to the **National Gallery of Art,** the building that is the closest to the Capitol in the string of big buildings on the north side. Since the Mall entrance to the Gallery is not accessible, push around to the front door on Constitution. Once inside you'll want to pick up a floor plan, a list of exhibits and a schedule of events for the day. You'll have quite a selection of things to see before dinner in the charming Gallery cafe, followed by the 7:00 P.M. concert in the garden court.

If the great masters ever dreamed of their paintings hanging in heaven, they probably envisioned them in a setting much like the National Gallery of Art. Your first impression when entering the exhibit level will probably be one of awe. Most people find themselves whispering as they come to the palatial marble rotunda from which the exhibit galleries radiate like spokes of a wheel. This grand room prepares one for the beauty of the paintings one is about to see, creating a mood that can only be called reverent.

Built to introduce Americans to European art, the National Gallery of Art includes such treasures as paintings by Rembrandt,

Vermeer, Ingres, Cézanne and Leonardo da Vinci. Not to be missed are the paintings on the Gallery's top twenty list. These include works by Raphael, Jan van Eyck, Fragonard, Poussin, Turner, Monet, Van Gogh, and Renoir.

In the spring of 1978 the Gallery opened its new East Building, which doubled exhibition capabilities. The innovative structure, designed to fit a triangular parcel of land, is in the shape of an isosceles triangle. Architect I.M. Pei conceived of three triangular towers, capped by a "space frame" skylight.

You'll get a sense of what this innovative architecture is about as you dine in the Gallery cafe or cafeteria. The subterranean dining facility, also designed by Pei, features a waterfall and an unusual skylighted ceiling. On the outdoor concourse one sees that the ceiling skylight is covered with four-sided glass projections. The closest comparison might be to an open-air deposit of stalagmites. The effect is fascinating.

After a tour of the Gallery, dinner, and contemplations of the fascinating architectural art forms created by Mr. Pei, you'll probably be ready for one of the Gallery's famous Sunday evening concerts. Head for the East Garden Court as early as possible so you can position yourself well for the 8:00 P.M. concert.

When your evening at the National Gallery of Art is over, head for the Constitution Avenue entrance and ask a guard to call a taxicab for you. As you taxi along Constitution Avenue look behind you for a glimpse of the Capitol and look for the Washington Monument on your left. Views of these two famous Washington, D.C., landmarks, lighted against the dark night sky, will round out a day of sightseeing pleasure in the nation's capital.

## TOUR 2

WHAT YOU'LL DO

- Visit the National Visitors' Center at Union Station.
- Self-tour of Capitol grounds.
- Visit Capitol, with conducted tour.

* Indicates restriction in time of use.
† All sites listed under "Restrooms" offer accessible facilities with wide stall doors and grab bars unless otherwise indicated.

- Visit Supreme Court, with conducted tour; lunch.
- Visit Library of Congress, with conducted tour.
- Dine at Hogates Restaurant.
- Make evening visit to the Jefferson Memorial.

HOW YOU'LL DO IT

- Push from your hotel to the Metro subway station, or take a cab to Union Station.
* - Subway Red Line to Union Station, Mass. Avenue and 1st Street N.E.
* - Subway from Union Station to Metro Center for transfer to Blue Line, then to Capitol South station, 1st Street and D Street S.E.
- Push two blocks along New Jersey Avenue to Capitol grounds.
- Enter Capitol from south side.
- Push two blocks from Capitol along East Capitol Street to Supreme Court, 2nd Street N.E. garage entrance.
- Push from Supreme Court two blocks to Library of Congress; enter beneath grand stairway.
- Cab from Library of Congress to Hogates Restaurant, 9th Street and Maine Avenue S.W.
- Cab from Hogates to hotel, with stop at Jefferson Memorial.

THINGS TO KNOW

- You'll need to buy a Metro subway fare card (see Getting Around section of this chapter for details).
- Best time for lunch at Supreme Court cafeteria is 11:30 A.M. or after 1:00 P.M.
- Tours of the Capitol and of Library of Congress are frequent, so exact timing of arrival is unnecessary.
- Hogates Restaurant open 11:00 A.M.–11:30 P.M. weekdays. No reservations taken.
- Jefferson Memorial is open until midnight, but for safety reasons ask cab driver to keep an eye on you or accompany you.
* - Subway may still run on weekdays only.

RESTROOMS †

- Capitol
- Supreme Court
- Library of Congress
- Hogates (accessible, but stalls only 26 inches wide)
- Union Station (accessible, but stalls only 26 inches wide)
- Metro subway station

Monday morning in the nation's capital is a bustling time. If you're staying downtown, you'll particularly note the activity. Head for your Metro subway station (see Getting Around for details on buying a fare card, using the handicapped-accessible entrance, determining how to get where you're headed).

**Union Station's National Visitors Center** serves as a prime source for travel information on the nation's capital and the rest of the country as well. Visitors are served at two desks dispensing information on Washington, D.C.: what to see, where to stay, and how to get around. In addition there is a special desk with specialized information for the handicapped visitor. So here you can gather the maps and information you'll need and at the same time see the famous old station, which was restored during the Bicentennial. Stop to see the audiovisual presentation on Washington, D.C., in the main hall, and enjoy a cup of tea or coffee at the cafe overlooking the busy station.

Continue from Union Station on the Red Line back to the transfer point at Metro Center, and take the Blue Line to the Capitol South station at First and D streets S.W. Ascending to street level, wheel along D Street to the right (east) to New Jersey Avenue; then, going slightly uphill, you'll see the **Capitol** two blocks ahead of you.

As you go, stop to enjoy the grounds, which contain over one hundred species of trees—one of the finest collections in the country. Look especially for the towering elm tree to the right of the Senate. It probably stood when the Capitol was only a blueprint. With patience you'll locate marked trees from thirty-three states, including such noteworthy specimens as a Japanese pine being raised as a bonsai, a cigarbox cedar from China, a twenty-foot redwood, a bald cypress, flowering dogwood and redbud trees, and eleven species of magnolia.

Feel free to ask questions of the many U.S. Capitol police you'll see along the way; they'll be able to direct you via the latest curb ramp.

Enter the Capitol at the north or south side and take the elevator up one floor to the Rotunda. You can join a thirty- to forty-five-minute tour that goes both to the Senate and House or just one. If you've written ahead (see "Planning Your Trip" for details) you'll also be able to spend some time in the House or Senate Gallery.

Plan on seeing the Capitol's main attractions, particularly the three newly-restored rooms completed in time for the Bicentennial. These are the Stuary Hall, which served as the House of Representatives until 1857; the Old Senate Chamber used by the Supreme Court for seventy-five years; and the original Supreme Court chamber restored to its 1860 look. Also see the Brumidi murals in the Senate wing, the Minton tiles from England that pave the way between the Senate Chamber and the Rotunda, the historical paintings in the Rotunda, and the Lincoln sculpture executed by a seventeen-year-old Virginia girl.

While you're in the area, you may want to follow the basement subway walkway to the Senate and visit the Senate Subcommittee on the Handicapped, located in room 10B of the Russell Office Building.

For lunch you can either push yourself the equivalent of two blocks on the underground Senate Subway walkway to the Senate Cafeteria, or leave the Capitol and push about two blocks through the parking lot and walkways to East Capitol Street and the **Supreme Court** with its fine ground-floor cafeteria. Enter via the garage on 2nd Street N.E. The Supreme Court cafeteria is one of the best in town, but because the Court staff gets priority, you must plan on lunching early (11:30 A.M.) or later (after 1:30 P.M.).

When court is in session (usually October to June, Monday through Thursday from 10:00 A.M. to noon, 12:30 to 2:30 P.M.) visitors may enter the chamber for a few minutes to hear an argument. Check with the attendant of the court. If the court is not in session, visitors may enter the chamber to hear a fifteen-minute talk.

From the Supreme Court, push back about two blocks to the **Library of Congress.** Considered the largest library in the world, this Italian Renaissance building, completed in 1897, houses some 85 million items, including books in all languages, films, records, tapes, maps, photos, and musical instruments.

Enter on the ground floor under the grand stairway, and check to see when the next forty-five-minute tour is leaving. On the tour or on your own, take the elevator up to the main floor to see the displays of such rare books as a Gutenberg Bible dating from 1455. See the display of important American documents, and go to the Visitors' Gallery to see the ornately decorated dome.

From the Library proceed by cab to **Hogates Restaurant** for a dinner of famous Chesapeake Bay softshell crab or other fresh fish. After dinner you may want to stop by the **Jefferson Memorial,** which is open each evening until midnight. Ask the cab driver to wait for you—better yet, invite him to accompany you—as you ascend the ramp on the west side of the Memorial. An internal elevator will get you to the base of the famed statue for a careful look at the 19-foot figure of Jefferson in dashing fur-collared great-coat. You'll want to read the four panels of his writings on the interior walls and look out over the Tidal Basin to the lights of the White House south portico. When you are in the White House the next morning you will reverse the view as you look from the window of the White House Blue Room to the Jefferson Memorial.

## TOUR 3

WHAT YOU'LL DO

- VIP tour of the White House.
- Tour of Lafayette Square.
- Lunch and tour of nationally famous Garfinckel's Department Store.
- Visit Museum of History and Technology for self-guided tour, movie, visit to museum shop, snack in cafeteria.
- Visit Museum of Natural History, take self-guided tour.
- Dine in or near hotel.
- Attend performance at Ford's Theatre.

* Indicates restriction in time of visit.

† All sites listed under "Restrooms" offer accessible facilities with wide stall doors and grab bars unless otherwise indicated.

HOW YOU'LL DO IT

- Cab from hotel to White House, East Executive Drive at Pennsylvania Avenue N.W., enter through east gate.
- Push four blocks from Lafayette Square to Garfinckel's Department Store, 14th and F streets N.W.
- Push two blocks from Garfinckel's to Metro Center subway station, 12th and G streets N.W.; or push four blocks down a slight hill to Pennsylvania Avenue and then along flat terrain to Constitution Avenue and 14th Street.
- \* • If by Metro, get off at the Smithsonian stop (Blue Line) and push across the Mall to the Museum of History and Technology.
- Push three blocks from the Museum of History and Technology to the Museum of Natural History, 10th Street and Constitution Avenue N.W.
- \* • Cab from Museum of Natural History to hotel or go by Metro subway if you wait until after 6:00 P.M. when the rush hour traffic has cleared somewhat.
- Cab from your hotel or from a restaurant to Ford's Theatre, 511 Tenth Street N.W.

THINGS TO KNOW

- You'll need tickets for the VIP White House tour (see Planning Your Trip for details).
- Garfinckel's Department Store opens at 10:00 A.M., the fifth-floor Greenbrier Restaurant at 11:00 A.M.
- All Smithsonian facilities open at 10:00 A.M.
- If you become a Resident Associate member of the Smithsonian, you can buy items in the museum shops at a 10 percent discount (see Planning Your Trip for details).
- Reserve a ticket for the evening performance at Ford's Theatre; advise them you're in a wheelchair.
- \* • Subway may still run on weekdays only.

RESTROOMS †

- Garfinckel's
- Museum of History and Technology
- Natural History Museum
- Metro subway station

Because the VIP tour of the **White House** begins at 8:30 A.M. in the fall, you might find this a good morning to order breakfast in your room. Then call a cab and get out at the east gate. You'll be admitted to the grounds and given a personally conducted tour of the residence, with stops at rooms not seen on the regular walk-through tours offered from 10:00 A.M. to noon, as well as the Kennedy garden used by the First Lady for entertaining.

On the VIP tour you'll have a peek in the White House library, stop in the China Room for a look at the official china of many first families, and visit the oval Diplomatic Reception Room, with its magnificent wallpaper of scenic wonders of America. Upstairs you'll visit the Green Room, furnished as a parlor in the style of Jefferson's time. Note the sofa that once belonged to Daniel Webster and the Monet painting given in memory of John F. Kennedy by his family.

In the Blue Room, note the life-size portrait of Jefferson, considered one of the two most popular paintings of him in the world; also see the pier table with mirror so ladies could adjust their long skirts. (From here you'll also look out to the Jefferson Memorial.)

In the Red Room the American Empire period is re-created with cerise silk walls and such furnishings as a sofa with a sphinx head, which belonged to Dolly Madison.

In the State Dining Room, notice Healy's portrait of Lincoln and the elaborate bronze-doré centerpiece that is considered one of the most historic treasures in the White House.

As you leave the famous north portico, stop to ask a fellow tourist to take your picture on the famous doorstep. Then wheel across Pennsylvania Avenue to Lafayette Square.

**Lafayette Square,** once part of the White House grounds, has been an orchard, a race track, trysting rendezvous, a site for demonstrations, and a favorite picnic spot for federal workers. Notice the statue of Lafayette on the southeast corner and the fine equestrian statue of Andrew Jackson in the center.

From a central location you can take a visual tour of the homes and buildings bordering this historic square. Beginning at the White House north portico tour clockwise to the gingerbread Old Executive Office Building and then along Jackson Place. The row of Federal-style town houses on Jackson Place is backed by the ten-story New Executive Office Building, designed with great care to complement the historic old houses. In this row toward the end, note the Decatur House, designed by Benjamin Henry Latrobe, the Capitol architect. Moving on to H Street, note the Hay-Adams Hotel, St. John's Church, and Parish House. This pretty yellow edifice was also built by Latrobe, who also designed the White House north portico across the square. The small church is so handy to the president's front door that every chief of state since John Adams has attended at least one of its services.

On the left border of the Square as you face the White House is the famed Cutts Madison House, where Dolly Madison lived. Daniel Webster lived just a few steps away, on the land where the imposing U.S. Chamber of Commerce Building now stands.

When you've had your fill of the historic sites, the flowers, trees, fountains, busy squirrels, and strollers, push back across Pennsylvania Avenue to 15th Street, then follow the slight incline down one block to F Street. **Garfinckel's,** the nationally famous department store, is at the corner of 14th and F streets. You may have a little time to kill before the store opens at 10:00, so roll around to see the many shops in this area, perhaps stopping for a cup of coffee at one of the drugstores or at the famous old Reeves Bakery on F Street between 12th and 13th streets.

After you've explored Garfinckel's and had lunch in the Greenbrier Restaurant on the fifth floor, have a cab called, push yourself, or board the subway at the Metro Center station and go to the **Museum of History and Technology** at 14th Street and Constitution Avenue.

You may choose not to go to Garfinckel's and head directly from the White House to the Museum instead. If so, the basement cafeteria, overlooking a sculpture garden, is a good place to lunch. Afterwards pick up the Museum map and listing of exhibits and check the times of the movies and special tours or demonstrations.

You'll have more than enough to choose from in this repository of fifty halls and bays filled with the country's most artfully displayed exhibits. Sections are devoted to music, scientific instruments, transportation, costumes, folk art, ceramics, stamps, coins, the armed forces, and much more. There is even a doll's house, and also an 1890s-style post office, an old-fashioned pharmacy, and a collection of merry-go-round animals. You won't want to miss seeing George Washington's false teeth, the Foucault Pendulum, the tattered remains of the original "star-spangled banner," and the hall of First Ladies' inaugural gowns. The Rehabilitation Discovery Corner, a newly opened niche at the museum, offers a dramatic view of devices to aid the handicapped.

At the **Natural History Museum** three short blocks away on Constitution Avenue you'll see more of the Smithsonian Institution collection. The fabulous collection includes specimens imaginatively displayed in areas devoted to archeology, anthropology, oceanography, geology, and zoology. Not to be missed are the dinosaurs, the Hope Diamond, the meteorites, a 92-foot model of a blue whale, the oldest known fossil in the world, dating back 3.1 billion years, and the Fenykovi elephant, the largest ever recorded, weighing in at 12 tons.

Instead of returning to your hotel, you could go by cab to Hammel's Restaurant, 416 10th Street, which is one block from the Ford's Theatre. But if you are returning to your hotel for a well-deserved rest, then consider having dinner in or near the hotel so you can get to the theater for the usual 7:30 P.M. curtain.

The **Ford's Theatre,** regarded as one of the most splendid theaters in the country when it opened in 1863, has been restored to look exactly as it did on the night Lincoln was shot. By using photographs taken just after the assassination, the National Park Service has recreated exact replicas of the original stage backdrop, the velvet stage curtains, the wallpaper, the cane-bottom chairs, and the Irish lace curtains, wallpaper, and furniture in the boxes.

You'll enter through the door on the far left, which has no stairs, and roll across the crimson-carpeted lobby into the orchestra section. You can remain in your wheelchair during the performance. From your vantage you'll see the president's box, draped with bunting. You may be able to picture Lincoln bowing to the crowds as the orchestra played "Hail to the Chief," and picture his sensitive face as he watched the drama unfolding on stage.

When you leave the theatre you can visually complete the saga of Lincoln's last hours as you look across the gaslit street at the Petersen House, where he died.

## TOUR 4

WHAT YOU'LL DO

- Lunch at the Patent Pending Cafe.
- Tour the National Portrait Gallery and National Collection of Fine Art.
- Visit the Foundry Mall in Georgetown with views of the C&O Canal.
- Dine at the Port o' Georgetown Restaurant.
- Entertainment at Blue's Alley.

HOW YOU'LL DO IT

- Push from hotel to Metro subway station.
* - Subway Red Line to Gallery Place station, 7th and G streets N.W.
- Push from station to National Portrait Gallery accessible entrance, 9th and G streets N.W.
- Cab from the Gallery to the Foundry Restaurant, 1050 30th Street.
- Push two-and-a-half blocks to Port o' Georgetown Restaurant, 1054 31st Street.
- Push a half block to Blue's Alley, 1073 Wisconsin Avenue.
- Cab from Blue's Alley to hotel.

THINGS TO KNOW

- Lunch served at Patent Pending Cafe from 11:00 A.M.–2:30 P.M.
- National Portrait Gallery and National Collection of Fine Art open 10:00 A.M.–5:30 P.M.
- Dinner served at Port o' Georgetown Restaurant from 5:00 P.M.–10:30 P.M.; no reservations necessary.
- Blue's Alley opens at 7:00 P.M.; admission charge $4.25 weekdays, $5 on weekends.
* - Subway may still run on weekdays only.

* Indicates restriction in time of use.
† All sites listed under "Restrooms" offer accessible facilities with wide stall doors and grab bars unless otherwise indicated.

RESTROOMS †

- National Portrait Gallery (men's, first floor; ladies', second floor)
- Foundry Shopping Center (restroom accessible, but stall doors are narrow)
- Metro subway station

More memories of Lincoln on this day of sightseeing when you visit the historic building where he held his second inaugural ball, now housing portraits and modern artworks. Then to the C&O Canal for a glimpse of mule-drawn barges, a look inside a new shopping center, and a ramble along charming old streets.

Begin your tour with an early lunch at the Patent Pending Cafe in the **National Portrait Gallery** and **National Collection of Fine Arts** complex. Both these parts of the Smithsonian Institution are housed in the old Patent Building.

Only the White House and the Capitol are older than this edifice, built by Washington Monument designer Robert Mills in 1840. The historic building was, until the 1940s, a repository of the inventions that made America the industrial leader of the world. Closed for ten years it was reopened in 1968 with its present collection. This grand old building served as the site of Lincoln's second inaugural ball and was a temporary hospital for soldiers during the Civil War. Inside you'll see a catalog of architectural styles: the Presidential Gallery, done in simple but rich Greek Revival style; the Sandstone Gallery, characterized by huge columns inspired by the ancient Greek island of Delos; the elegant Model Hall, a late-Victorian wonderland of Pompeii mosaic tiles, stained glass windows, ornate brass-railed balconies, and marble pillars.

To reach this building, go by Metro subway Red Line to Gallery Place at 7th and G streets N.W. You can roll two blocks along G Street to the accessible entrance to the Portrait Gallery, but with just a little more energy you'll find the route around the front of the old Patent Building more interesting. Head down 7th Street to F Street and go along F Street to the corner of 9th. You'll find yourself in a landscaped plaza bright with flowers and fountains. This is one of the "Streets for People" projects of the District government, designed to improve downtown Washington. The fountains were designed for participation, and they seem to have achieved their purpose. You'll probably see children dashing through the low jets of water and hanging happily around the spraying fonts. Stop to look at the unique audiovisual display show inside huge open-ended domes. If you have a question or need a map, ask at the information kiosk.

As you push along 9th Street to the accessible entrance, you'll also see Library Place, a second part of the project. This one features a flowing water fountain that becomes a babbling brook as it travels through stone channels under white-flowering trees. Note the D.C. Public Library, which was designed by Mies van der Rohe.

Enter the old Patent Building through the garage on 9th and G streets to avoid the twelve-step entrance. The two art collections are separated by a courtyard filled with trees, benches, and sculpture, an ideal place for an outdoor lunch, which can be purchased at the **Patent Pending Cafe.** Chili, quiche, soup, sandwiches, apple pandowdy topped with whipped cream are among the offerings.

After lunch you can get serious about the two collections. On display in the Portrait Gallery are formal portraits, sculpture, and photographs of famous Americans. Note the charming miniature of George Washington painted at Mt. Vernon for Martha, the matching portraits of John Adams and Thomas Jefferson, and the famous William Draper portrait of John F. Kennedy.

At the National Collection of Fine Arts you'll have a survey of American painting, sculpture, and crafts with the emphasis on the contemporary. The collection occupies two wings and includes more than 12,000 works, among them the paintings of George Catlin, famed for his canvases of American Indians and Indian life.

When you're ready to leave, exit the way you came in and meet the taxicab you ordered.

Get out at the **Foundry Restaurant** and you'll be on the banks of the old C&O Canal. Before the days of railroads, this waterway was the main means of moving wheat, coal, and occasionally whiskey between the capital and the cities to the northwest. One of its key promoters and investors was George Washington, who envisioned the canal linking Washington with the country's interior.

The narrow artery stretches for 184 miles to Cumberland, Maryland. As in the nineteenth-century days when mules pulled work scows along its sycamore-lined banks, so today twentieth-century mules pull a modern replica of an old canal barge along the timeless waterway. You'll probably see the barge tied up at the lock just opposite the restaurant.

You can enjoy the canal scene from inside the Foundry Restaurant through picture windows that open onto the water and park. Next to the restaurant is the **Foundry Mall,** a modern red brick shopping complex built around some of the original red brick walls and oak trusses of the old Duvall Foundry.

Inside you can browse through the bookstores, art galleries, garden and food shops. An elevator links the mall level with a downstairs level built around an intriguing black fountain and pond. Of particular interest in this shopping center are the marine paintings at the **Atlantic Gallery,** the African art at **Brady & Jones,** and the Oriental furniture at **Jean Morrow Ltd.**

If you have an able friend along, you may want to explore Georgetown, which is barren of curb cuts and is a bit rocky in places. With someone to assist you, you can tour the side streets and the main promenade, M Street. At 30th Street and M, your friend can push you across the street to the **Old Stone House,** built in 1765 and neatly restored and outfitted with modest furniture and utensils. A pretty garden to the side of the house makes an ideal place for people-watching. As you continue the tour, enjoy the windows and look into some of the shops, which sell everything from antiques and modern furniture to Indian clothing and green plants. For a snack, try the cappuccino at **Cafe de Paris,** a phyllo-wrapped cheese pastry at **Ikaros,** or pizza at the **Black Olive.**

Although much of Georgetown is hilly, with rough streets and few curb cuts, you can go a short distance on your own. Wheel up 30th Street, turn left onto M Street, and turn toward the canal at 31st Street. A driveway about midblock connects with a driveway across the street, permitting you to get to another shopping complex, the Port o' Georgetown Square.

If you don't decide to buy moveable feasts to enjoy beside the canal, enjoy the canal scene from the porch of the **Port o' Georgetown Restaurant,** at 31st and M streets. You can sip a drink outdoors and then dine within on a salad you make yourself, hot bread, and a choice of entrees.

After dinner, drop by **Blue's Alley,** just a few feet from Port o' Georgetown. This famous jazz club features such top entertainers as Carmen McCrae, Oscar Peterson, and Stan Getz.

Conclude your day with a cab ride along Pennsylvania Avenue, around Washington Circle, and through the quiet downtown area to your hotel.

## TOUR 5

### WHAT YOU'LL DO

- Tour Washington Cathedral, with a visit to the herb shop.
- Visit the National Zoo and lunch beside the duck pond.
- Refreshments at Kramerbooks.
- Windowshop along Connecticut Avenue.
- Dine at the rooftop Chaparral Restaurant in Rosslyn.

### HOW YOU'LL DO IT

- Cab from your hotel to Washington Cathedral, Wisconsin and Massachusetts Avenue N.E., northwest entrance near Security Station.
- Cab from the Cathedral to the National Zoological Park, Connecticut Avenue N.W., west of Calvert Street.
- Cab from Zoo to Kramerbooks & Afterwords Cafe, 1517 Connecticut Avenue N.W. (one high step at entrance).
- Push across the street to subway elevator entrance, Connecticut Avenue and Q Street N.W.
* - Subway to hotel.
- Cab from hotel to Chaparral Restaurant in the Marriott–Key Bridge Hotel, Rosslyn, Virginia.

### THINGS TO KNOW

- Washington Cathedral tours hourly from 10:00 A.M, lasting about forty minutes.
- National Zoo open daily 9:30 A.M.–6:00 P.M. in the summer, 9:00 A.M.–4:30 P.M. the rest of the year. Free.

---

\* Indicates restriction in time of visit.

† All sites listed under "Restrooms" offer accessible facilities with wide stall doors and grab bars unless otherwise indicated.

- Chaparral Restaurant serves dinner weekdays from 6:00 P.M. to 10:00 P.M. Reservations advised.
* • Subway may still run on weekdays only.

RESTROOMS †

- National Zoo, in Police Station and in Delicate Hoof Stock buildings
- Washington Cathedral (accessible restrooms, but stalls only 26 inches wide)
- Metro subway station

Beyond the busy downtown streets, the monuments and cobblestone streets of Georgetown, lies a city of gracious apartment houses, leafy residential streets, and quiet parks.

You'll see today the sometimes exotic elegance of Washington's Embassy Row, the beauty of our nation's only Gothic cathedral, and the furry treasures in your own national zoo. You begin with a cab ride to the Washington Cathedral. Ask your driver to go to the Cathedral via Dupont Circle and Massachusetts Avenue so you'll have a chance to see part of Embassy Row. Dozens of embassies and chanceries line the broad tree-lined avenue. At its elegant heart lies Sheridan Circle surrounded by a marvellous group of early twentieth-century mansions. In few areas of America are there better concentrations of pre-World War II wealth. As you enjoy this driving tour look for the embellishments of the Beaux Arts styles, the influences of the Frank Lloyd Wright School, Gothic and French details. If your interest is architecture, this may be your sightseeing highpoint.

Of particular interest is the showy Indonesian Chancery housed in an ornate mansion built by the father of Evelyn Walsh MacLean, the owner of the Hope Diamond. Across the street at 2107 Massachusetts Avenue, note the charming stone elephants outside the Embassy of India. Continuing up Massachusetts Avenue you'll pass the Embassy of Ireland, the Embassy of Turkey with its wealth of eighteenth-century European detail and Frank Lloyd Wright influences, and the Embassy of the United Republic of Cameroon, noted for its sixteenth-century French design.

Look for the handsome grounds surrounding the Embassy of Japan, the mosaic tiles around the entrance to the Embassy of

Iran, and the British Embassy with its statue of Churchill.

Just before arriving at the Cathedral, you'll see the Naval Observatory, where the vice-presidential family has its official residence.

The **Washington Cathedral** (often called the National Cathedral) reigns atop the highest point of land in the District. Many consider the fourteenth-century Gothic-style edifice to be the most beautiful cathedral in America. Begun in 1907 when President Theodore Roosevelt laid the cornerstone, its towers of St. Peter and St. Paul should be completed in 1984.

The complex includes grounds that ramble over Mount Saint Albans, lovely gardens, schools, and an herb and spice shop. If you join the hourly tour you'll see some fine French and English architectural details within and some of the most glorious stained glass windows in the country. The new Rose Window was unveiled in 1976. Following the tour, roll over to the spice and herb shop for a sniff of woodruff or mint, perhaps buying some seeds as a memento of your visit.

Continue next to the **National Zoological Park,** a short cab ride away. The zoo, although completely accessible with all exhibits ramped, is somewhat hilly. It's a good place to have a friend to push you along. But if not, you can still see something of this fine zoo on your own.

Look at the map as you enter the grounds to get your bearing in this large park where some 2400 animals reside, including about thirty kinds of animals almost extinct in the wilds. A must for most people are the giant pandas—the only ones in the Western Hemisphere—given as a gift by the People's Republic of China. You'll also want to see the first white tiger in our hemisphere and the big outdoor flight cage. Newest addition is the unique Beaver Valley exhibit, with above- and below-water views of such creatures as bush dogs, beavers, seals, and sea lions.

Lunch in the zoo cafeteria, or buy hot dogs and soft drinks from vendors and lunch beside the ponds where migrating ducks join the resident exotics.

Plan on leaving the zoo before rush hour traffic, about 3:30, and return to Connecticut Avenue, getting out of the cab at **Kramerbooks & Afterwords Cafe.** In this bright and airy store ideal for browsing, you'll have the rare opportunity to consider your purchases closely as you enjoy apple juice, coffee, or some tidbits from the charming cafe that adjoins the bookshelves.

From Kramerbooks you can reach the subway elevator entrance, which is directly across the street, by going up and down curbs or, if you prefer, roll one short block south to the intersection of Connecticut Avenue and 19th Street where you'll find curb cuts. By going the longer way you'll have the chance to do some interesting window shopping along this fashionable shopping haven.

Should you be the hearty type or have assistance, you may want to explore more of Connecticut Avenue or enjoy the music and people in busy Dupont Circle, just a few feet and several curbs away.

After your subway ride back to your hotel and time to read or rest, thoughts of dining while viewing the capital may tantalize. If so, call for a reservation and head by cab a few miles across the Potomac River to Arlington and the penthouse **Chapparel Restaurant** in the Marriott Hotel. Here, overlooking the Potomac River, the bridges and monuments of the capital, you can enjoy such classics as prime rib, lobster, and filet mignon, or try the fascinating Chapparel Combination: black bean soup, crab crêpe, sauteed shrimp, medallion of beef, salad, and Black Forest cake.

As you dine you'll see the monuments you have already visited and get a sneak preview of the Kennedy Center for the Performing Arts and the Lincoln Memorial—both highlights on your agenda for the following day.

## TOUR 6

WHAT YOU'LL DO

- Return visit to one of the Smithsonian museums.
- Lunch at the Smithsonian or in your hotel.
- Tour Lincoln Memorial.
- Tour Arlington Cemetery.

\* Indicates restriction in time of visit.
$ ___ /$ ___ indicates adult/child admission fees.
† All sites listed under "Restrooms" offer accessible facilities with wide stall doors and grab bars unless otherwise indicated.

- Cruise on the Potomac River.
- Tour the State Department.
- Tour, have dinner, and see performance at the Kennedy Center.

### HOW YOU'LL DO IT

* • Subway Blue Line to Smithsonian station, Independence Avenue and 12th Street S.W.
- Cab tour from Smithsonian to Lincoln Memorial (use east entrance), then to Arlington Cemetery, then to Potomac Boat Tours dock, southwest of Lincoln Memorial on Ohio Drive S.W.
- Cab from boat dock to Department of State, 2200 C Street N.W.
- Push with assistance three long blocks or cab from Department of State to Kennedy Center.
- Cab from Kennedy Center to hotel.

### THINGS TO KNOW

- Smithsonian opens at 10:00 A.M.
- Cost of cab trip to Lincoln Memorial, waiting time, and continuation to Arlington Cemetery or Potomac Boat Tours dock can be negotiated at hourly rate.
* • Potomac Boat Tours leave hourly Tuesday–Sunday from 11:00 A.M.–3:00 P.M. after Labor Day; from April 1–Labor Day, 10:00 A.M.–9:00 P.M. Call 548–5010 to doublecheck times. Tour costs $3/$1.50.
* • Subway may still run on weekdays only.
- VIP tours of Department of State Reception Rooms at 3:30 P.M. Arrangements must be made ahead (see Planning Your Trip for details).
- Tickets for Kennedy Center performances should be reserved ahead (see Planning Your Trip for details), but it's possible to buy tickets on the day of the performance.
- La Grande Scene open from noon to 2:30 P.M., 5:30 P.M. to after last curtain. The Gallery and the Promenade open 11:30 A.M.–8:00 P.M.

RESTROOMS †

- Smithsonian Institution
- Lincoln Memorial
- Kennedy Center

Begin your final day of sightseeing in Washington with a return visit to the Smithsonian, a morning of shopping around your hotel, or take a cab to the offices of the President's Committee on Employment of the Handicapped, 1111 20th Street N.W., to pick up literature and greet some of the staff.

Lunch at the cafeteria in the Museum of History and Technology, outside this same building on the rear patio overlooking the Mall, or in or near your hotel.

After lunch, call a cab, and when the cabbie arrives let him know that you'd like to hire the cab by the hour. You'll not only save money by doing this but also will be assured of getting a cab without waiting in an area where cabs are not plentiful. In one hour you should be able to make a brief stop at Lincoln Memorial and also drive across Memorial Bridge for a tour of Arlington Cemetery.

En route to the Lincoln Memorial you'll pass the Washington Monument and the Bicentennial addition, the Constitution Gardens, a graceful expanse of 2600 trees, winding paths, and a large island-centered lake. Beyond, through fringes of trees, is the reflecting pool that mirrors the Washington Monument and fronts the famous steps of the **Lincoln Memorial.**

If the Capitol is the heart of Washington, her soul is the Lincoln Memorial. Since its completion in 1922 the Lincoln Memorial has drawn to its cool marble steps those who dream and who pray. Because Lincoln was the Great Emancipator, the Memorial has become a living symbol for the oppressed. The blacks, the poor, the war-weary have come to draw inspiration from the seated figure of Lincoln that fills the interior of this temple to the spirit.

As you approach the monument, which was patterned after the Parthenon, you'll glimpse the 19-foot sculpture between the columns. Inside, at its feet, you can observe the expressive face from different directions, seeing the determined Lincoln from head on, the smiling Lincoln from the right, and the frowning Lincoln from the left. Considered one of the great sculptures of the world, it is also one of the most reproduced, since it has appeared on more than 80 million pennies. The National Park Service gives fifteen-minute tours throughout the day during which you'll learn the details of its execution. On your own you'll want to read the Gettysburg Address and the Second Inaugural Address, which are inscribed above the figure. Note above the inscriptions the murals portraying emancipation and unity.

At **Arlington National Cemetery** handicapped visitors can get a pass from the Visitors' Center so that they can drive or be driven on the roads that are otherwise closed to automobiles. The most popular sight, the Kennedy grave site, can't be seen by the average wheelchair traveler since the trail to it is steep. If you have a friend to assist you, this is the time to invite him along; otherwise ask your cab driver to push you—he may be willing to unofficially. Even without a close look at the Kennedy grave site, the drive through Arlington Cemetery is interesting, affords lovely views of Washington, and permits a close look at the Custis-Lee Mansion, officially known as Arlington House.

Don't miss the chance to see the hourly changing of the honor guard at the Tomb of the Unknown Soldier.

If you're visiting the Cemetery with a friend you might want to take advantage of the free Tourmobile passes available from the Cemetery Visitors' Center. With the pass, a wheelchair user and an able friend may board the shuttle (but there is no ramp, so a mobilely handicapped person must be lifted aboard) for a guided tour of the grounds.

With only a little wristwatch-watching you should be able to get back across Memorial Bridge in time to board the 2:00 P.M. **Potomac Boat Tours** cruiser for more sightseeing. The boat, which leaves from the dock southwest of the Lincoln Memorial on Ohio Drive, plies the Potomac River between Georgetown and Hains Point. From the stern, where wheelchairs are accommodated, you'll see the capital city from a new perspective while enjoying a panorama of islands, bridges, and boats. The fifty-minute tour features a running narrative by a tour guide who points out such sights as the Kennedy Center, Georgetown University, Roosevelt Island, and the Lady Bird Johnson fountain at the tip of Hains

Point. Towards the end of the tour, ask one of the attendants to call a taxicab for you so that when you arrive back at the dock it will be waiting or about to appear.

Then off you go a few blocks (but steep uphill blocks) to the **Department of State,** where you will enjoy the VIP tour of the reception rooms (see Planning Your Trip for details on arranging for this tour). With a group of other guests you'll see the rooftop rooms where the U.S. government entertains kings, queens, sheiks, and maharanis. The eighteenth-century drawing and reception rooms are filled with America's finest antiques and art objects. The John Quincy Adams state drawing room, said by many to be the most beautiful room in America, contains a cache of priceless highboys, lowboys, chests, desks, and chairs, all gleaming under a glory of crystal chandeliers and sconces from a Lisbon palace. The well-versed guides have stories to tell about almost every object, thus bringing American history into delightful new perspective.

After the hour-long tour, stop by the government bookstore in the State Department, one of many open to the public around Washington.

From the State Department you probably will find the three block ramble to the Kennedy Center pleasant and easy. Roll along 23rd Street to the corner of E, cross the street, and continue down 23rd Street past the Columbia Plaza apartment complex and the Pan American Health Organization with its dramatic fountains. Turn the corner at Virginia Avenue and proceed down the street as far as you can go and then follow the curve past People's Life Insurance to the path that cuts through a green stretch of gardens to the doors of Kennedy Center.

The $70 million **Kennedy Center,** completed in 1971, is as grand as it is innovative. Few structures offer more ideal accessibility for the wheelchair traveler or more to see and do—and not just theatrical performances. In addition to the obvious, people also go to Kennedy Center to enjoy the spectacular rooftop views, to dine, and to people-watch. If you have theater tickets for the evening (see Planning Your Trip for details), great, otherwise make your selection from the postings and see what's available. You'll be choosing from a musical comedy, ballet, or opera being staged in the Opera House, a concert in the Concert Hall, a play in the

Eisenhower Theater (he's the president who initiated the project of building a theatrical center), or a movie in the American Film Theater.

But before the performance you'll have plenty of time to explore the Center. Consider taking the free conducted tour offered by the National Park Service; ask at the desk near the first of the two main entrances when the next one leaves. Then, with this tour or on your own, look for the remarkable treasures given by many countries of the world to make the Center so special: the Aubusson tapestries representing the Creation in the South Gallery were a gift from Australia; the Austrians presented the crystal chandelier in the Opera House; there is a porcelain relief from Denmark in the Concert Hall lobby; there are twenty planters from India in the Grand Foyer; black and white wool rugs on the Roof Terrace Galleries are Moroccan.

Circle the outdoor rooftop promenade for breath-taking views of the capital and the river.

For dinner choose between the elegant **La Grande Scene** restaurant, the **Promenade** cafeteria and outdoor terrace, or the **Gallery Cafe.** One Washington restaurant reviewer has called the Center's Black Forest cake "superb"—you probably will too.

Before enjoying a theatrical performance join the pre-theater throng in the lobby, admire the sculpture of President Kennedy, and treat yourself to a glass of champagne, served in the lounge areas.

Following the performance, if the night is clear, take a last look at Washington from the rooftop terrace, or stop for a libation before signaling one of the cabs that wait outside the Center. By the time you leave, the most hectic portion of the after-theater crowd will have hurried on and you in your cab will see the quiet streets of the capital and enjoy a final evening view of the Washington Monument as you head back to your hotel.

### Other Accessible Attractions

B'nai B'rith Exhibit Hall, 1640 Rhode Island Avenue N.W.
Corcoran Gallery of Art,* 17th Street and New York Avenue
    N.W. (service entrance on E Street)

Daughters of American Revolution Museum,* 1776 D Street N.W. (D Street entrance)

Franciscan Monastery,* 1400 Quincy Street N.E. (accessible from eastside door)

Lightship *Chesapeake*, 1200 Ohio Drive S.W. (steep ramp 25 inches wide)

Museum of African Art,* 316 A Street N.E. (two steps)

National Aquarium, Commerce Department, 14th and Constitution Avenue N.W. (ramped entrance)

National Archives, 7th Street and Constitution Avenue N.W. (ramped entrance at 8th and Pennsylvania)

National Arboretum, Bladensburg Road and R Street N.E.

National Geographic Society,* 17th and M streets N.W. (call for portable ramp: 296–7500)

National Historical Wax Museum, 333 E Street S.W. (one step)

National Shrine of the Immaculate Conception, 4th Street and Michigan Avenue N.E.

Philips Collection, 1612 21st Street N.W. (one step)

Renwick Gallery,* 17th Street and Pennsylvania Avenue N.W. (call 381–5811)

U.S. Botanical Gardens, 1st and Canal Street S.W. (ramp at northwest corner)

Washington Monument, Mall at 15th Street N.W.

INTRODUCING

*Rollin' On* adviser, wheeler Diane Lattin

*Title:* Editor, *Disabled USA*, President's Committee on Employment of the Handicapped

*Telephone number:* (202) 653–5010

*Hometown:* Washington

*Favorite tourist site:* Lincoln Memorial

*Hidden corner:* Constitution Gardens, on Constitution Avenue between the Lincoln Memorial and the Washington Monument

*Rendezvous:* Mayflower Hotel lobby

*Offbeat restaurant:* Rumor's

* Call before going

*Place for music:* The Dubliner
*View:* from the Lincoln Memorial
*Natural wonder:* Great Falls in nearby Maryland
*Museum:* National Air and Space Museum
*Ramble:* along the C & O Canal in Georgetown
*Non-tourist destination:* the offices of the President's Committee
    on Employment of the Handicapped (visitors welcome)
*Off-beat experience:* riding the subway
*Traditional restaurant:* Maison des Crepes
*Low-cost restaurant:* Scholl's Cafeteria
*Ice cream shop:* Baskin-Robbins on Wisconsin Avenue or Nature's
    Way for frozen yogurt
*Reading suggestion: All the President's Men* by Bob Woodward
    and Carl Bernstein
*Place to get a wheelchair repaired:* Abbey Rents
*Tips on having a great time in Washington:* Go to zoo and feed
    marshmallows to the bears; they do wonderful things for
    marshmallows. Go to The Dubliner and feed Guinness to an
    Irishman; Irishmen do wonderful things for Guinness.

# 13

# Other Cities

## Boston

A unique city with top historic sites, but also with narrow, hilly streets and old buildings flanked by stairs. Some of the historic buildings are accessible, but because they're often on hills, you'll have to reach them by car or cab, with not much chance to wheel between destinations. All possible, particularly if you have assistance.

Included among the accessible historic sites are these:

Old South Meeting House
Old City Hall
Paul Revere House
Old North Church
Harrison Gray Otis House

Boston also has its relatively flat areas good for rolling around. Among the best areas are the waterfront extension of the Heritage Trail, the plaza and malls surrounding Prudential Center, and the beautifully restored Quincy Market next to Faneuil Hall. You'll have a nice choice of things to do and see on your own once away from the historic hill area. Sightseeing could include these accessible possibilities:

Prudential Tower Skywalk
Boston Common
John Hancock Observation Tower

Massachusetts Horticultural Society
Public Garden
Isabella Stewart Gardner Museum
Museum of Science
Museum of Fine Arts

The ideally situated Sheraton Boston Hotel, 39 Dalton Street at Prudential Center, offers rooms especially designed for the physically disabled. From it you can roll to the Prudential Building with its observation deck and to numerous restaurants and entertainment attractions. Among the other hotels with wheelchair-accessible rooms:

Howard Johnson's, 57 Park Plaza
Howard Johnson's, 320 Washington Street
Howard Johnson's, 575 Commonwealth Avenue
Holiday Inn–Somerville, 30 Washington Street
Holiday Inn–Peabody, rts. 1 and 128
Holiday Inn–Burlington, Middlesex Turnpike and Wheeler Road
Holiday Inn–Woburn, 19 Commerce Way

A surprising number of restaurants in this city are accessible, including one that actually offers restroom facilities for the handicapped, the Stella Restaurant, 74 East India Row.

For a complete listing of restaurants and other tourist information as it relates to the wheelchair traveler, write for *A Guide to Boston for the Handicapped*, c/o The Rehabilitation Council, United Community Services, 14 Somerset Street, Boston, Massachusetts 02108. Information and a map of Boston are available from the Greater Boston Convention and Tourist Bureau, 900 Boylston Street, Boston, Massachusetts 02115.

### Denver

Beautiful, friendly, curb-ramped Denver, a great place for the wheelchair traveler, particularly if he or she is on a tour of Colorado or of the West. This city makes a good one- or two-day stop when you're on your way somewhere else, but it probably doesn't offer the tourist enough for a single-destination vacation. With so much within easy driving range, there's no reason to linger over-long in Denver, but while you're there there are some choice things to enjoy.

A pleasant day can be spent touring the U.S. Mint, visiting the Denver Art Museum and Historical Museum, and then exploring Larimer Square, a historic renovation. A second day can continue nicely with a drive to the Denver Zoo and Museum of Natural History, and can be concluded with a twilight view, concert, and picnic supper at Red Rock Park.

Wheelchair-accessible restaurants abound, including such downtown favorites as:

Boston Half Shell
Fisherman's Cove
The Golden Ox
Le Bistro
Le Profil
Mario's
Quorum
Sperte's Laffite
Top of the Rockies

Local wheelers claim to have one of the most accessible hotels in the west, Stouffer's Denver Inn, near the airport at 32nd and Quebec streets. Others with especially designed wheelchair rooms include:

El Patio Motel, 8400 East Colfax
Holiday Inn–Downtown, 15th and Glenarm Place
Holiday Inn–North, 4849 Bannock Street
Holiday Inn–Airport, 4040 Quebec
Holiday Inn, 1475 South Colorado Boulevard
Regency Inn, 3900 North Elati

For more information on the accessible attractions of the city, write for *A Guidebook to Denver for the Handicapped*, c/o the Sewall Rehabilitation Center, 1360 Vine Street, Denver, Colorado 80206. Tourist literature is available from the Convention and Visitors Bureau of Denver, 225 West Colfax, Denver, Colorado 80202.

## Miami

Again and again reports come in that Miami is not that great for wheelchair travelers. It may help to know that both the city and county governments are working on the problem. Many of the municipalities that make up Dade County, of which Miami is part, now have their own advisory groups counseling their governments on matters concerning the handicapped. Nearly $300,000 is allocated for cutting ramps into existing curbs, and $100,000 for making Miami park facilities accessible.

The wheeler who goes to Miami will find at least five hotels offering rooms especially designed for the physically disabled. They are:

> Holiday Inn, 1170 N.W. 11th Street
> Holiday Inn, 679 N.W. 79th Street
> Holiday Inn, 1111 South Royal Poinciana Boulevard
> Howard Johnson's, 16500 N.W. Second Avenue
> Howard Johnson's, 12210 Biscayne Boulevard

Rich in tourist sights, the Miami area offers a wealth of things to see and do. Among the accessible possibilities:

- Parrot Jungle, a garden of exotic orchids and cactus where tropical birds fly, monkeys play, and alligators laze
- Eleventh-century Spanish monastery brought to the United States by William Randolph Heart and reassembled stone by stone
- The tribally owned Tiger Miccosukee Indian Village, where you see alligator wrestling and Indian crafts
- Miami Museum of Science, with its exhibits of Florida wildlife, coral reef fish, and Tequesta Indian relics
- Donnin's Antique Arms and Gun Museum, a large collection of weapons and armor from the past and present
- Miami Beach Conservatory and Gardens, showing tropical horticulture from all over the world
- Bayfront Park, a wide concrete promenade fronting the bay, winding among acres of greenery

The Marine Stadium for boat races, the West Flagler Kennel for dog racing, the Orange Bowl for football, and the Miami Auditorium for boxing all are accessible.

For information on sightseeing options, hotels, and entertainment facilities, write for the *Wheelchair Directory* put out by the Florida Paraplegic Association, 1366 Terrace, Miami Beach, Florida 33139.

Also write for the general tourist literature dispensed by the Miami Beach Tourist Development Authority, 555  17th Street, Miami Beach, Florida 33139.

## New Orleans

The problem with New Orleans is that the French Quarter has uncut curbs and few driveways, so the wheeler who's unassisted may have trouble. However, there is a positive development, the offering of scheduled tours by Medicab of Metropolitan New Orleans. The usual high cost of Medicab becomes realistic when shared with a group. Four tours began operating in September 1977: one of the city, a brunch and jazz tour, a riverboat cruise, and a tour to the Moorish-Spanish Longue Vue Gardens. Transportation is also available from the New Orleans International Airport.

For information write to Medicab of Metropolitan New Orleans, 53 Smithway, Gretna, Louisiana 70053, or call (504) 367–7720.

Holiday Inn and Howard Johnson's both offer rooms especially designed for the physically disabled:

> Holiday Inn, Airport-West, 6401 Vets Memorial Boulevard
> Holiday Inn–Downtown, 330 Loyola Avenue
> Howard Johnson's–Airport, 6401 Vets Memorial Boulevard
> Howard Johnson's–Downtown, 330 Loyola Avenue
> Holiday Inn–Superdome, 1111 Gravier Street

Although not offering specifically designed wheelchair rooms these hotels in the French Quarter may be possibilities:

> Chateau Motor Hotel, 1001 Chartres (bathroom door 30 inches)

Downtowner Motor Inn, 541 Bourbon Street (bathroom door 22 inches)

Holiday Inn–French Quarter, 124 Royal (bathroom door 28½ inches)

Prince Conti Motor Hotel, 830 Conti Street (bathroom door 24 inches)

Some of the most famous of the French Quarter restaurants are accessible, including:

Antoine's Restaurant, 713 St. Louis Street

Arnaud's, 813 Bienville Street (one step)

Brennan's, 417 Royal Street

All three of the big jazz spots can accommodate wheelchairs; each has one step at the entrance:

Al Hirt, 501 Bourbon Street

Pete Fountain's, 800 Bourbon Street

Preservation Hall, 726 St. Peter Street

The Jackson Square area, with the St. Louis Cathedral and St. Anthony Garden, has been made into a pedestrian mall for lots of good rambling, and on certain hours Royal Street and Bourbon Street also turn into non-auto malls.

As for sightseeing there are some good accessible restored homes, museums, and parks, including the Gallier House, a faithfully restored 1860s residence; the masterpiece of historical authenticity, the Musée Conti Historical Wax Museum; and the New Orleans Museum of Art in the City Park.

The Easter Seal Society has just come out with a new edition of its *Guide to New Orleans for the Physically Disabled*, which you can obtain by requesting it from them at 3939 Veterans Boulevard, Metairie, Louisiana 70002.

For information on the city write to the Tourist and Convention Commission, 334 Royal Street, New Orleans, Louisiana 70130.

## Phoenix

Phoenix, with its neighboring suburb Scottsdale, is considered by wheelers to be one of the most accessible cities. The flat terrain and the facilities for its large retirement population make it a good place for the wheelchair traveler.

Several hotels offer rooms especially designed for the physically disabled:

Camelback Sahara Motor Hotel, 2935 West Clarendon Avenue

Del Webb's Hotel, 100 West Clarendon Avenue

Hyatt Regency, 111 West Monroe

Among the top accessible restaurants are:

China Doll, southwest corner Seventh Avenue and Osborn Road

Golden Eagle Restaurant, 201 North Central

Hermosa Inn, 5532 North Palo Cristi Road

Los Olivos Resort Hotel, 202 East McDoweil Road

Navarre's, 52 East Camelback Road

Playboy Club, 3033 North Central Avenue

As for things to see and do, Phoenix Civic Plaza offers an accessible theatre and Scottsdale offers the Center for the Arts. Sightseeing can include the accessible Phoenix Zoo, the Tropical Gardens, Encanto Park, and the Desert Botanical Gardens. The Heard Museum, with its collection of primitive arts from Arizona Indian cultures, is partially accessible.

The *Directory of Barrier-Free Buildings* can be obtained from the Easter Seal Society, 703–6 North First Street, Phoenix, Arizona 85004. Information on the city is available from the Convention and Visitors Bureau, 2701 East Camelback Road, Phoenix, Arizona 85016.

## Seattle

Outstanding! If this book featured a ninth city, it probably would be Seattle. Even though Seattle is known as a city of hills, some of the best sightseeing lies in the relatively flat areas like downtown, the historic Pioneer Square, and the site of the Seattle World's Fair with its current $20 million remodeling program.

By early 1979 the city's electric trolley system will include 109 new vehicles with wheelchair lifts. There are three hotels offering disabled units: the Hilton Hotel Downtown, the TraveLodge Sea-Tac, and the Washington Plaza Hotel.

At least twenty-eight of the accessible restaurants also offer restrooms especially designed for wheelchair use!

In addition, the city is involved in a vast curb ramp program. One local wheeler who is also a spokesman for the city's Department of Human Resources says, "Without bragging, I'd have to say that Seattle—except maybe for transportation—is the most accessible major city in the country."

For the detailed *Access Seattle* guidebook, write to the Easter Seal Society, 521 Second Avenue West, Seattle, Washington 98119. General information on the city is available from the Seattle–King County Convention and Visitors Bureau, 1815 Seventh Avenue, Seattle, Washington 98101.

See the chapter Travel Information Sources that follows for a city by city listing of guides for the disabled traveler.

# *14*

# Travel Information Sources

## Travel Publications for the Mobiley Disabled

### General

"Access National Parks:
A Guide to the National Parks for the Handicapped," $3.50
    Consumer Information Center
    Pueblo, Colo. 81009

"A List of Guidebooks for Handicapped Travelers," 5th edition
    President's Committee on Employment of the Handicapped
    Washington, D.C. 20210

"Consumer Rights for Disabled Citizens" (includes a section on travel), $2
    Dept. of Consumer Affairs
    80 Lafayette St., New York, N.Y. 10013

"Travel Tips for the Handicapped"
    Consumer Guides, United States Travel Service
    U.S. Dept. of Commerce, Washington, D.C. 20230

Easter Seal Access Guides
    Information Center
    National Easter Seal Society
    2023 West Ogden Ave.
    Chicago, Ill. 60612

## By Transportation Mode

"Access Amtrak"
Public Affairs, Amtrak
400 N. Capital St. N.W., Washington, D.C. 20001

"Access Travel: Airports"
Consumer Information Center
Dept. 619-F, Pueblo, Colo. 81009

"Air Travel for the Handicapped"
TWA Sales Dept.
2 Penn Plaza, New York, N.Y. 10010

"Handicapped Driver's Guide"
American Automobile Assn.
(check the address of your local office in your phone book)

"Helping Hand Service for the Handicapped"
Greyhound Lines
Greyhound Tower, Phoenix, Ariz. 95077

"Highway Rest Areas for Handicapped Travelers"
The President's Committee on Employment of the Handicapped
Washington, D.C. 20210

### Guidebooks for the Mobiley Disabled

ALASKA
**Anchorage**
"Anchorage Guide for the Physically Handicapped" (1975)
Anchorage Rehabilitation Assn.
910 MacKay Bldg., 338 Denali St.
Anchorage, Alaska 99501

ARIZONA
**Phoenix**
"Directory of Barrier-Free Buildings" (1975)
Easter Seal Society of Arizona
702–706 N. 1st St.
Phoenix, Ariz. 95504

ARKANSAS
**Hot Springs**
"A Guide to Hot Springs for the Handicapped"

Garland County Easter Seal Society for Crippled Children and Adults, Inc.
2801 Lee Avenue
Little Rock, Ark. 72205

CALIFORNIA

**Beverly Hills**
"Around the Town With Ease—A Guide for the Physically Limited Person"
Junior League of Los Angeles
Beverly Wilshire Hotel
9500 Wilshire Blvd. at Rodeo Dr.
Beverly Hills, Calif. 90212

**Los Angeles**
"Around the Town with Ease"
Junior League of Los Angeles
6333 West Thire St.
Los Angeles, Calif. 90043

**Oakland**
"A Guide to Oakland and Parts of Berkeley for the Physically Disabled and Aging"
Easter Seal Society
2757 Telegraph Ave.
Oakland, Calif. 94609

**Palo Alto**
"Getting Around in Palo Alto" (1976)
City of Palo Alto
Office of Community Relations
250 Hamilton Ave.
Palo Alto, Calif. 94301

**San Diego**
"A Step in Time—San Diego Guide for the Handicapped" (1977)
Junior League of San Diego
House of Hospitality, Balboa Park
San Diego, Calif. 92109

**Sacramento**
"A Guide Book to Sacramento for the Physically Handicapped and Aging"
The Easter Seal Society for Crippled Children

and Adults of Sacramento
3205 Hurley Way
Sacramento, Calif. 95825

**San Francisco**
"Guide to San Francisco for the Disabled"
(1976)
Easter Seal Society
6221 Geary Blvd.
San Francisco, Calif. 94121

COLORADO

**Denver**
"A Guidebook to Denver for the Handicapped" (1976)
Commission on the Disabled
619 S. Broadway
Denver, Colo. 90223

**Fort Collins**
"Open Doors for the Handicapped"
Chamber of Commerce
2716 E. Mulberry
Fort Collins, Colo. 80521

**Loveland**
"Guide to Open Doors in Loveland, Colorado: Cultural, Educational, Recreational and Service Facilities"
Easter Seal Society of Larimer County
2716 East Mulberry
Fort Collins, Colo. 80521

CONNECTICUT

**New Britain**
"Your Key to New Britain" (1977)
Chamber of Commerce
127 Main St.
New Britain, Conn. 06052

**Waterbury**
"Access Waterbury: 1977"
Easter Seal Rehabilitation Center of Greater Waterbury
22 Tompkins St.
Waterbury, Conn. 06708

DELAWARE

**Georgetown**
"Welcome Handicapped Visitors" (1977)
Delmarva Easter Seal Rehabilitation Center
204 E. North Street
Georgetown, Del. 19947

**Rehoboth**
"Welcome Handicapped Visitor" (1977)
Chamber of Commerce
Convention Hall
Rehoboth, Del. 19971

**Wilmington**
"A Guide to Northern Delaware for the Disabled" (1974)
Easter Seal Society for Crippled Children and Adults of Mel-Mar
2705 Baynard Blvd.
Wilmington, Del. 19802

"As It Is"
Delaware Paralyzed Veterans
1601 Kirkwood Highway, Room 13
Wilmington, Del. 19805

DISTRICT OF COLUMBIA

**Washington**
"Access Washington" (1977)
Information Center for Handicapped Individuals, Inc.
1413 K St., NW
Washington, D.C. 20005

FLORIDA

**Jacksonville**
"Guide to the Handicapped—Jacksonville" (1976)
Easter Seal Society
1056 Oak St.
Jacksonville, Fla. 32204

**Lower Pinellas County**
"Accessibility" (1977)
Easter Seal Rehabilitation Center
7671 US Highway 19
Pinellas Park, Fla. 33565

**Manatee & Sarasota Counties**
"Guide for Physically Handicapped (Manatee & Sarasota Counties)" (1972)
Sarasota County Society for Crippled Children and Adults
401 Braden Ave.
Sarasota, Fla. 33580

**Miami**
"Wheelchair Directory"
Florida Paraplegic Assn.
1366 Terrace
Miami Beach, Fla. 33139

**Orlando**
Orlando Area Tourist Trade Assn.
P.O. Box 15492
Orlando, Fla. 32809

**Sarasota**
"Guide to Physically Handicapped Manatee and Sarasota Counties" (1972)
Happiness House Rehabilitation Center, Inc.
401 Braden Ave.
Sarasota, Fla. 33580

**Tampa**
"Guide to the Tampa Area for the Physically Handicapped" (1976)
Easter Seal Society
2401 E. Henry Ave.
Tampa, Fla. 33610

GEORGIA

**Albany**
"Guide for the Handicapped to the Greater Albany Area" (1975)
The Southwest Georgia Area Easter Seal Rehabilitation Center
1906 Palmyra Rd.
Albany, Ga. 31701

**Atlanta**
"Getting About Atlanta"

Georgia Easter Seal Society
Atlanta, Ga. 30309

HAWAII

**Maui**
"Maui Easter Seal Society—Guide for the Handicapped"
Maui Unit
National Easter Seal Society for Crippled Children and Adults, Inc.
P.O. Box #183
Kahukui, Hawaii 96732

ILLINOIS

**Chicago**
"Access Chicago" ($1)
401 E. Superior St.
Chicago, Ill. 60611

"Access North Suburban Chicago" (1977) ($1)
League of Women Voters of the Deerfield Area
P.O. Box 124
Deerfield, Ill. 60015

**Springfield**
"Building Access Guide for the Handicapped and Aging" (1972)
Eileen McCune, Chairman
Altrusa Club of Springfield
623 East Adams St.
Springfield, Ill. 62706

INDIANA

**Indianapolis**
"Navigation Unlimited in Indianapolis" (1972)
Marion County Muscular Dystrophy Foundation
615 North Alabama St.
Indianapolis, Ind. 46204

IOWA

**Des Moines**
"A Guidebook to Des Moines for the Handicapped"
Alpha Omicron Alpha Chapter
Alpha Chi Omega
Des Moines, Iowa 50306

**Dubuque**
"Handicapped Guide to Accessible Places"
Project Access Dubuque
P.O. Box 122
Dubuque, Iowa 52001

KANSAS

**Topeka**
"Facilities Directory: A Guide to Accessible Establishments" (1976)
Division for the Disabled
City Hall, Room 54
Topeka, Kan. 66603

**Wichita**
"A Guide for the Disabled of Wichita" (1975)
($1)
Easter Seal Society of Kansas, Inc.
3701 Plaza Dr.
Topeka, Kan. 66609

KENTUCKY

**Ashland**
"A Guide to Ashland for the Handicapped"
Kentucky Society for Crippled Children
233 East Broadway
Louisville, Ky. 40202

**Louisville**
"A Guide to Louisville for the Handicapped" (1967)
Kentucky Society for Crippled Children
233 East Broadway
Louisville, Ky. 40202

LOUISIANA

**New Orleans**
"A Guide to New Orleans for the Physically Disabled" (1978)
Easter Seal Society
P.O. Box 8425
Metairie, La. 70011

**Shreveport**
"A Guide to Facilities in Shreveport and Bossier City" (1964)
Community Council Office

1702 Irving Pl.
Shreveport, La. 71101

MAINE

"Maine Guide for the Handicapped and Elderly Traveler"
Governor's Committee on Employment of the Handicapped
32 Winthrop St.
Augusta, Me. 04330

MARYLAND

**Baltimore**
"Ready, Set, Go"
The Baltimore Central Maryland League
1111 East Cold Spring La.
Baltimore, Md. 21239

MASSACHUSETTS

**Boston**
"A Guide to Boston for the Handicapped"
Rehabilitation Council
United Community Services
14 Somerset St.
Boston, Mass. 02108

"Access to Boston in '76"
The Easter Seal Society of Massachusetts
37 Harvard St.
Worcester, Mass. 01608

**Fall River**
"The Greater Fall River Area Handbook for the Handicapped"
Fall River Chamber of Commerce
332 Milliken Blvd.
Fall River, Mass. 02721

**Springfield**
"A Guide to Springfield for the Physically Disabled and Aging"
The Easter Seal Society for Crippled Children and Adults of Massachusetts, Inc.
30 Highland St.
Worcester, Mass. 01608

**Worcester**
"Wheeling through Worcester" (1973)

Easter Seal Society for Crippled Children and Adults of Massachusetts, Inc.
37 Harvard St.
Worcester, Mass. 01608

MICHIGAN

**Flint**
"A Guide to Flint for the Handicapped" (1972)
Easter Seal Society
1420 W. 3rd Ave.
Flint, Mich. 48504

**Pontiac**
"Rights and Information for Persons With Handicaps" (1976) ($2.50)
Oakland County Easter Seal Society
1105 North Telegraph Rd.
Pontiac, Mich. 48053

MINNESOTA

"Easy Wheelin' in Minnesota" (1976)
Robert Peters
#1 Timberglade Rd.
Bloomington, Minn. 55437

MISSISSIPPI

**Jackson**
"A Key to Jackson for the Physically Limited" (1976)
Mississippi Easter Seal Society
P.O. Box 4958
Jackson, Miss. 39216

MISSOURI

**Columbia**
"Access in Columbia" (1976)
College of Home Economics
University of Missouri–Columbia
239 Stanley Hall
Columbia, Mo. 65201

**St. Louis**
"St. Louis Has It A to Z For The Handicapped" (1975)
The Easter Seal Society, St. Louis Region
4108 Lindell Blvd.
St. Louis, Mo. 63108

NEBRASKA

**Omaha**
"A Guide to Omaha for the Handicapped"
(1967)
Easter Seal Society
Box 1420 W. Om St.
Omaha, Neb. 68114

NEW MEXICO

"A Guide for the Handicapped"
New Mexico Society for Crippled Children
and Adults, Inc.
1803 Central Ave., S.E.
Albuquerque, N.M. 87100

NEW YORK

"Vacationland New York State" (1977)
Easter Seal Society
2 Park Ave.
New York, N.Y. 10016

**New York**
"The New York City Guide"
Easter Seal Society
2 Park Ave., Suite 1815
New York, N.Y. 10016

"Access New York" (50¢)
Institute of Rehabilitation Medicine
400 East 34th St.
New York, N.Y. 10016

**Schenectady**
"Access to Capital Lands" (1976)
Junior League of Schenectady
Box 857
Schenectady, N.Y. 12309

**Syracuse**
"See Syracuse—A Guide for the Handi-
capped" (1968—revision forthcoming)
Easter Seal Society
1103 State Tower Building
Syracuse, N.Y. 13202

**White Plains**
"Handy Guide for the Handicapped" (1976)
Westchester Society for Crippled Children and
Adults, Inc.
171 East Post Rd.
White Plains, N.Y. 10601

NORTH CAROLINA    **Chapel Hill**
"Guide to Chapel Hill"
Town Administration Bldg.
306 N. Columbia St.
Chapel Hill, N.C. 27514

OHIO    **Akron**
Akron Area Guide for the Handicapped
Junior League for Akron
929 W. Market St.
Akron, Ohio 44313

**Canton**
"Guide to Canton for the Handicapped"
Goodwill Industries and Rehabilitation Clinic
408 9th, S.W.
Canton, Ohio 44314

**Cincinnati**
"Greater Cincinnati Guidebook for the Han-
dicapped" (1977)
The Hamilton County Easter Seal Society
7505 Reading Rd.
Cincinnati, Ohio 45237

**Dayton**
"A Guide to Dayton for the Handicapped"
(1969)
Junior League of Dayton
Dayton, Ohio 45402

**Toledo**
"A Guide to Toledo for the Handicapped"
Toledo Area Chamber of Commerce
218 Huron St.
Toledo, Ohio 43604

"Guide for the Physically Handicapped to Buildings and Facilities in Toledo, Ohio" (1977)
Toledo Society for the Handicapped
630 West Woodruff Ave.
Toledo, Ohio 43624

OREGON

### Oswego Lake
"A Guide for the Handicapped"
Oregon Society for Crippled Children and Adults, Inc.
4343 S.W. Corbett Ave.
Portland, Ore. 97201

PENNSYLVANIA

### Erie
"Accessibility Guide" (25¢)
The Task Force
645 East 23rd St.
Erie, Pa. 16503

### Delaware County
"Guide to Delaware County for the Handicapped" (1976)
Delaware County Easter Seal Rehabilitation Center of the Society for Crippled Children and Adults
468 North Middletown Rd.
Media, Pa. 19063

### Philadelphia
"Guide to Philadelphia for the Handicapped" (1976)
Mayor's Office for the Handicapped
City Hall Annex, Room 427
Philadelphia, Pa. 19107

### Pittsburgh
"A Guide to Pittsburgh for the Handicapped"
Open Doors for the Handicapped
1013 Brintell St.
Pittsburgh, Pa. 15201

### State College
"A Guide to Downtown State College for the

Disabled and Aged" (1976)
The Easter Seal Society for Crippled Children
and Adults of Centre and Clinton Counties
1300 South Allen St.
State College, Pa. 16801
FREE: to aged or handicapped in Centre &
Clinton Co.
PRICE: $1.00 out of Centre and Clinton
Counties

RHODE ISLAND

**Providence**
"Guide to Rhode Island for the Handicapped"
Crippled Children and Adults of Rhode Island, Inc.
333 Grotto Ave.
Providence, R.I. 02906

SOUTH DAKOTA

"Wheelchair Vacationing in South Dakota"
(1976)
Division of Tourism
Joe Foss Building
Pierre, S.D. 57501

**Black Hills and Badlands**
"Wheelchair Vacationing in the Black Hills
and Badlands of South Dakota"
Guide Booklet for the Handicapped
Black Hills, Badlands and Lakes Association
Box 539
Sturgis, S.D. 57785

TEXAS

**Dallas**
"A Guide to Dallas for the Handicapped"
The Professional Group of The Junior League
of Dallas, Inc.
5500 Greenville Ave.
Dallas, Tex. 75206

"Access Dallas '77"
Texas Easter Seal Society for Crippled Children and Adults
4429 North Central Expressway
Dallas, Tex. 75205

**Gonzales**
"Wheeling Around Texas"
Former Patient Association
Texas Rehabilitation Association
P.O. Box 58
Gonzales, Tex. 78625

**Houston**
"Accessibility Guide to Houston for the Handicapped" (28¢)
Texas Institute of Rehabilitation and Research
1333 Moursund Ave.
Houston, Tex. 77030

**San Antonio**
"A Guide to San Antonio for the Handicapped"
Easter Seal Society
2818 S. Pine St.
San Antonio, Tex. 78210

VIRGINIA

**Roanoke Valley**
"Guide for the Handicapped and Aging"
Secretary, Mayor's Committee on Employment of the Handicapped
P.O. Box 61
Roanoke, Va. 24002

WASHINGTON

**Seattle**
"Access Seattle" (1977)
Easter Seal Society
521 2nd Ave. West
Seattle, Wash. 98119

**Spokane**
"Guide to Spokane for the Handicapped"
Easter Seal Society
West 510 Second Ave.
Spokane, Wash. 99204

WEST VIRGINIA

"West Virginia Travel for the Handicapped"
WV Rehabilitation Association
Structural Barriers Program

1427 Lee St. East
Charleston, W.Va. 25301

**Wheeling**
"Wheeling through Wheeling" (1974)
Wheeling Ohio Co. Planning Commission
Room 305, City County Building
1500 Chapline St.
Wheeling, W.Va. 26003

WISCONSIN

**Milwaukee**
"A Guidebook to Milwaukee for the Handicapped"
The Easter Seal Society for Crippled Children
and Adults of Milwaukee County, Inc.
5225 W. Burleigh St.
Milwaukee, Wis. 53210